In the Arms
of Morpheus

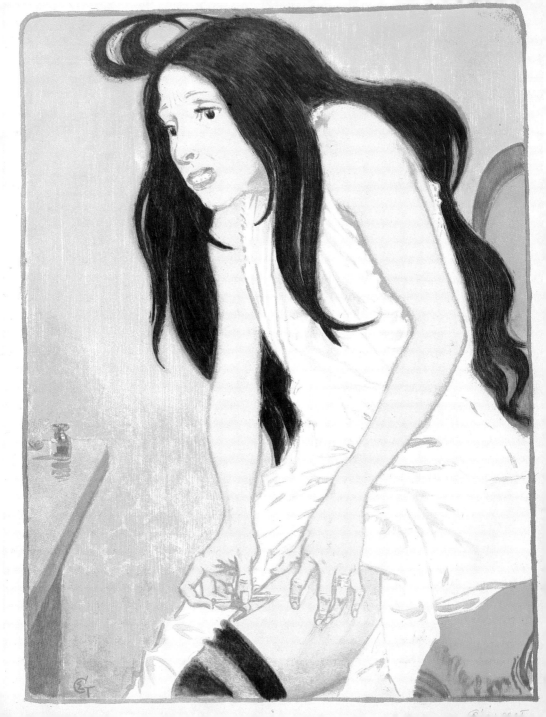

In the Arms of Morpheus

THE TRAGIC HISTORY OF LAUDANUM, MORPHINE, AND PATENT MEDICINES

Barbara Hodgson

FIREFLY BOOKS

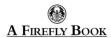

A FIREFLY BOOK

Published by Firefly Books (U.S.) Inc. 2001

First Printing

U.S. CATALOGING IN PUBLICATION DATA
  (Library of Congress Standards)

Hodgson, Barbara.
    In the arms of Morpheus : the tragic history of morphine, laudanum and patent medicines / Barbara Hodgson. – 1st ed.
        [160] p. : ill. (some col.) ; cm.
    Includes bibliographical references and index.
    Summary : Social history of the use of opium derivatives.
    ISBN 1-55297-538-X   ISBN 1-55297-540-1 (pbk.)
    1. Opium – Social aspects. 2. Opium – History. 3. Hallucinogenic drugs – Social aspects. 4. Hallucinogenic drugs – History. 5. Narcotic habit – Social aspects.   I. Title.
    362.29/ 3   21   2001

First published in the United States in 2001 by
Firefly Books (U.S.) Inc.
P.O. Box 1338, Ellicott Station
Buffalo, New York 14205

Originated and simultaneously published in Canada by Greystone Books, Vancouver.
Edited by Nancy Flight
Design by Barbara Hodgson/Byzantium Books
Printed and bound in Hong Kong by C&C Offset

Image acknowledgements are adjacent to specific images. All uncredited images are from Byzantium Archives. Images without attribution are from unknown sources or by unknown artists. Every effort has been made to trace accurate ownership of copyrighted text and visual material used in this book. Errors or omissions will be corrected in subsequent editions, provided notification is sent to the publisher.

Frontispiece: Morphinomaniac, colour lithograph by Eugène Samuel Grasset, 1897. Courtesy Philadelphia Museum of Art. Purchased with the SmithKline Beckman (now Beecham) Fund for the Ars Medica Collection. Photo by Graydon Wood, 1997

Facing page: Dr. J. Collis Browne's Chlorodyne ad from 1917.

Running head: Poppy adapted from engraving by Constant Le Breton in *Consolata: Fille du Soleil* by Henry Daguerches, Paris: Lemercier, 1928.

The names of medicines containing opium, morphine or heroin can be found running along the bottom of each page, beginning with the introduction. Although there are over three hundred names, the list is by no means exhaustive. Some medicines may be in dispute, but if a medicine has been found in a formulary with opium listed in the contents it has been put on this list. A single date means that I found one reference to the drug for the year indicated; a range means that I found multiple references within the years shown. The country shown is where the drug originated or likely originated. US = United States, GB = Great Britain, Aus. = Australia, Can. = Canada

Contents

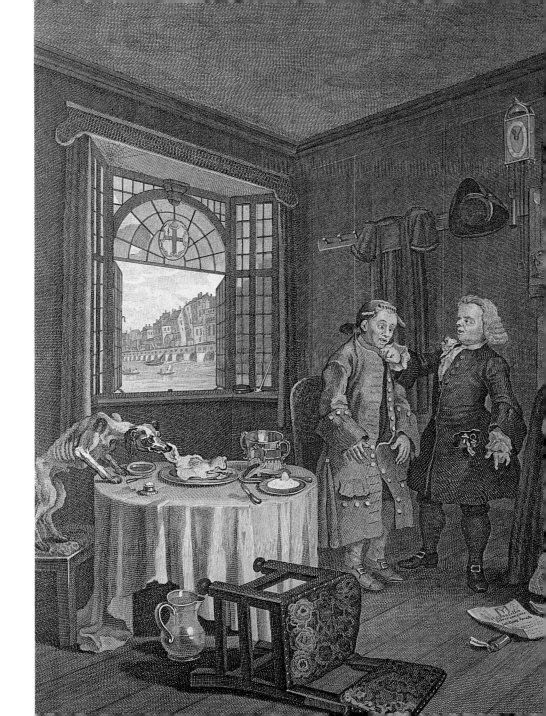

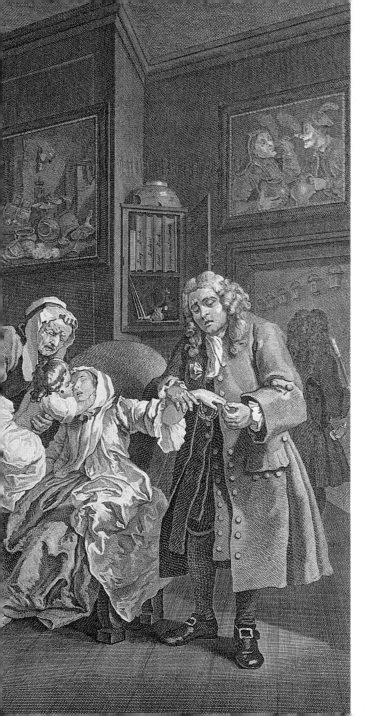

Marriage à la Mode, Plate VI, "The Suicide of the Countess." The last panel of William Hogarth's scathing series on the life of English aristocracy shows the lifeless Countess Squanderfield, an empty bottle of laudanum at her feet, being kissed by her long-neglected child. She had just read of the hanging of her husband for the murder of her lover, Counsellor Silvertongue. Engraved in 1745 from the original c. 1743 painting. A detail of the laudanum bottle is shown below.

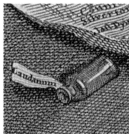

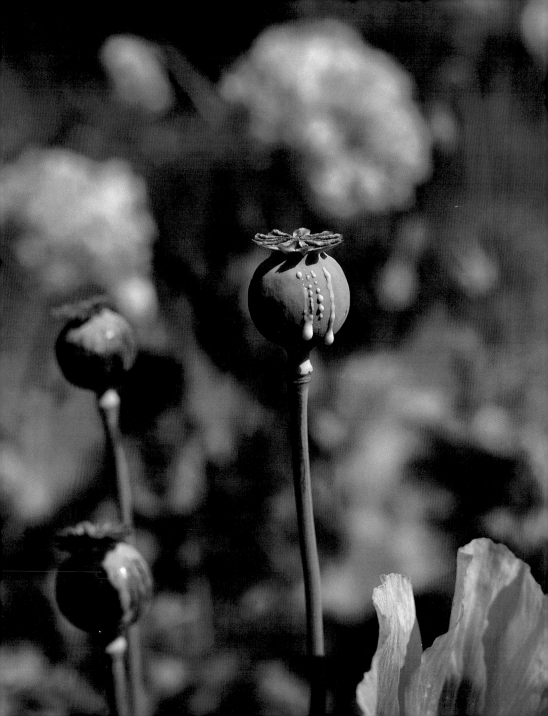

Introduction

IN THE ARMS OF MORPHEUS

Sleep had a thousand sons, and of that number
He made the choice of waking Morpheus.—Ovid, *Metamorphoses*

Ode to the Poppy, 1792

"Hail, lovely blossom!—
thou can'st ease,
The wretched victims of
disease;
Can'st close those weary eyes,
in gentle sleep,
Which never open but to
weep;
For, oh! thy potent charm,
Can agonizing pain disarm;
Expel imperious memory
from her feat,
And bid the throbbing heart
forget to beat."
—Charlotte Smith[1]

Papaver somniferum. Ripe pods of the
opium poppy, scored and exuding sap,
which will dry into opium.

*H*ow fitting it is that Morpheus, the god of dreams, should inspire the naming of morphine, one of the most powerful sleep-inducing, dream-making drugs ever known. Ovid immortalized Morpheus as somnolence personified in *Metamorphoses*, and from then on he was used as a metaphor for repose. The only son of Somnos, the god of sleep, Morpheus was able to take the shape of a man, thus tying into the Greek word *morphē*, meaning having form. The image of a being who steals over us to close our eyes and bring us rest has had a number of incarnations, including Somnos, Hypnos, Brother of Death and even good-natured Mr. Sandman.

Morphine is opium's principal alkaloid, or active ingredient, and is present in all opium, regardless of where it has been grown or how it has been processed. Opium, the dried sap of the poppy *Papaver somniferum*, consists of over two dozen alkaloids; of these, only morphine and codeine have medicinal significance. Without morphine, and to a lesser extent codeine, opium's effectiveness would be nearly nonexistent, as would its addictiveness; few substances on this earth provoke dependency as thoroughly as morphine.

Opium in its raw state is dark brown, bitter tasting and gummy. It can be eaten, mixed in flavoured beverages or made into tinctures, syrups, pills or plasters. Or it can be processed for

Adam's Cough Cure (US 1897); Allen's Lung Balsam (US 1902); Antikamnia & Heroin Tablets (US 1890–1900s);

smoking. Morphine in its isolated form is a white crystallized salt that can be dissolved or melted for use in medicines that are swallowed or injected.

Whereas opium has been recognized for its medicinal attributes for at least 2500 years, morphine was not isolated and identified until the first decade of the 1800s. Before that time, making and prescribing opium medicines took some guesswork because the morphine content in opium varies so much—from 3 to 17 per cent. Although the substitution of pure morphine for opium produced medicines that were more powerful and reliable, opium continued to be an important ingredient throughout the nineteenth century.

Opium—and thus morphine—was the key component in an astounding number of medicines, both reputable and quack. One of the most popular of these was laudanum, or tincture of opium, a potent mixture of wine, opium, saffron and cinnamon. The medicine of choice of nineteenth-century writers, artists and ordinary folk, not only was laudanum legitimate, it had an allure all of its own. But there were hundreds of cure-alls that were unmitigated shams. These were the infamous patent medicines, which, contrary to their name, were rarely patented, had little or even negative medicinal value and were made from anything with a therapeutically bad taste or a scientific or exotic name. Opium surfaced in countless elixirs created between 1700 and 1906, because it gave the semblance of a cure. And, as a plus for manufacturers, it left customers with a yen for more.

All opium medicines, whether they are made from opium or refined morphine, are used against pain, coughing or diarrhoea. It is now known that morphine, and thus opium, inhibits pain and produces calm by attaching itself to receptors on certain nerve

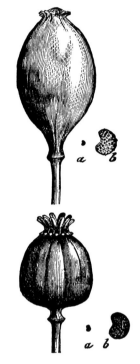

Capsules and seeds (*a:* natural size and *b:* magnified) from two varieties of the opium poppy. *Top:* from the black poppy (*Papaver somniferum* var. *nigrum*); *bottom:* from the white poppy (*Papaver somniferum* var. *album*). From Alfred Stillé and John Maisch, *The National Dispensatory.* Philadelphia, 1880, 1056.

A true panacea? In 1908, opium and morphine were prescribed for the following ailments: threatened abortion, alcoholism, aneurism, angina pectoris, irritated bladder, boils, bronchitis, cancer, catarrh, chilblains, cholera, chordee, intestinal colic, renal colic, convulsions, cough, delirium, delirium tremens, diabetes, diarrhoea, dysentery, earache, epilepsy, erysipelas, typhoid fever, gallstones, gastralgia, goitre, chronic gonorrhoea, gout, haematemesis, haemoptysis, haemorrhoids, headache, hiccough, hysteria, acute inflammation, rheumatism, kidney disease, lumbago, acute mania, measles, melancholia, mumps, neuralgia, acute peritonitis, phthisis, pleuritis, pneumonia, pruritus (itching), pyrosis, sciatica, sprains, stomach ulcers, strangury and whooping cough.[2]

cells in the brain. These receptors already produce similar but natural narcoticlike substances known as endorphins, sort of homemade pain relievers. So the body, accustomed to its own, albeit not as effective, form of painkiller, recognizes and welcomes the morphine molecules. Once established in the brain, morphine controls pain, coughing, vomiting, euphoria and states of wakefulness. It also works separately on the gut, freezing the muscles in the intestines and thereby controlling bowel movements. Altogether morphine can provoke flushing, sweating, constipation, itchiness, nausea, sleepiness, restlessness, anxiety and shortness of breath.

A quantity of opium sufficient to dull the agony of a toothache will usually produce little more than a mild numbness followed by a deeper than usual sleep along with a slight costiveness in a person who has no need of pain relief. A larger dose may produce nausea or an overwhelming sleepiness or inexplicable restlessness. Those unaccustomed to taking morphine have a higher risk of overdosing than those who take it habitually. The more one is accustomed to taking morphine, the larger the quantity required just to feel normal. An overdose, in any of morphine's forms, including raw opium, can result in death.

Accidental overdoses are rarer than morphine's other side effects, which are universal and almost immediate. To some, the most distressing is the speed with which constipation sets in, followed by even more distressing rapid relief when the drug is stopped. And although opium usually induces sleep, that sleep is often disturbed, the restlessness carrying over into the waking hours. In some, morphine causes insomnia. As well, the appetite tends to fall off, and though the drive for sex at first increases, this is temporary; interest and ability soon plummet. These conditions disappear once the opium is cleared from the body.

A fascinating question, for which there seems to be no set answer, is how long does it take to become addicted to opium? Most observers agree that it depends on the frequency and strength of the doses, the way it is administered, the severity of the ailment for which it has been prescribed and the ease with which the individual develops dependencies. An addiction to laudanum, which came in varying strengths, takes longer to develop than an addiction to morphine injections. Opium in the former instance is diluted in three ways: it is raw opium, which has an average morphine content of 10 per cent; it is added to another ingredient, wine; and once swallowed, it is mixed with gastric juices. With morphine injections, 100 per cent morphine is introduced into the body and travels directly to the brain without any dilution along the way.

Morphine puts the patient at ease while—it is hoped—a cure is underway, but if the malady has not been dealt with by the time the patient stops taking the drug, the symptoms return. In the meantime, the patient has been experiencing a sense of well-being but needs increasing amounts of morphine to maintain that euphoria; in other words, the patient develops a tolerance to the drug. When attempts are made to stop using it, the intense craving for the drug that develops brings its own physical suffering. Whether it's called morphinism, *morphinomanie* or *morphiumsucht*, it's the same thing, an addiction, or an insatiable desire for morphine. Fortunately, today, since other, nonaddictive drugs are available, morphine is limited to short-term use and to palliative care, and dependence on it through medical application is rare.

Opium! "Dread agent of unimaginable pleasure and pain! I had heard of it as I had heard of manna or of ambrosia, but no further. How unmeaning a sound was opium at that time! what solemn chords does it now strike upon my heart! what heart-quaking vibrations of sad and happy remembrances!"—Thomas De Quincey[3]

A word on heroin

Appearing in 1898, the discovery of Bayer Company chemist, Heinrich Dreser, heroin's role in medicine was similar to morphine's. Also known as diacetylmorphine, it was initially used to treat respiratory conditions. Even more addictive than morphine, its use for coughs and colds was discontinued early in the 1900s, though it was used to control pain until relatively recently, especially in Britain and Australia.

(GB 1820–80); Bayer's Heroin Hydrochloric (Germany 1898); Beecham's Cough Pills (GB 1897–1909); Bertha C. De

Dr. Judas "The opium inquisitor brings out the rack and stretches the victim upon it without delay."[4]

Climbing the ladder of opium "My capability for mental exertion all through this period was something incredible; and let me say here that one of the most fascinating effects of the drug in the case of an intellectual and educated man is the sense it imparts of what might be termed intellectual daring: add to this the endowments of a strong frame, high animal spirits, and on such an one, opium is the ladder that seems to lead to the gates of heaven. But alas for him when at its topmost rung!"— Anonymous[5]

Never confuse the opium-smoker with the opium-eater. Quite different phenomena.—Jean Cocteau

My previous book *Opium: A Portrait of the Heavenly Demon* considered popular attitudes towards opium smoking up to 1930, before and just after narcotic possession became illegal throughout the West. This book examines attitudes towards medical preparations of opium during the same time period. Although medicinal opium was used and abused around the world, my emphasis is on Europe and North America.

The seemingly indiscriminate use of medicinal opium in the past is a complex subject, at times incomprehensible to our current sensibilities. Why did all of those doctors prescribe such addictive medicines? Why did all of those mothers drug their children? It's easy to take a critical point of view, but we'd be on rocky ground if we were to censure this behaviour. Before the twentieth century, those who were ill had little choice but to turn to a substance such as opium. At least three conditions paved the way for this situation. First, opium was a vital means of coping with cholera, dysentery and tuberculosis, diseases borne of horrific living conditions such as those of the Industrial Revolution, because it reduced the physical manifestations of the diseases—for example, diarrhoea and coughing. Second, many diseases were incurable; opium eased the pain brought on by these ailments. And last, because opium was effective, available and cheap, those who distrusted or couldn't afford medical help diagnosed and treated their ailments themselves. In cases where the medical profession was consulted, many doctors knew little more than their patients and so prescribed opium for the same reasons.

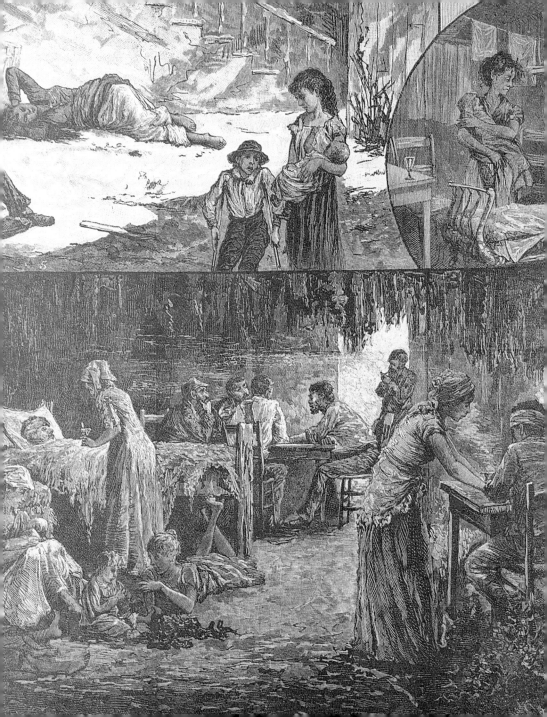

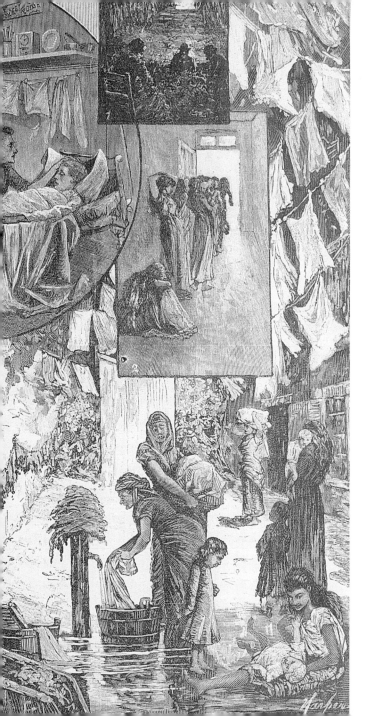

Poverty "In this class of houses it is the young who suffer most . . . ill nourished, ill cared for, they fall in great numbers before the pitiless assaults made on their young lives from every corner of their wretched homes. If we are shocked that in this Christian city there should be such helpless victims, we can not deny that those who die earliest are the happiest."— *Harper's Weekly*[6]

Tenement-House Life, New York. *Harper's* frequently tackled social issues such as poverty, intemperance, idleness and corruption. This drawing by W. St. John Harper commemorates the visit of Mayor Grace of New York to the city's most notorious slums. *Harper's Weekly*, 15 October 1881, 696.

There is but one all-absorbing want, one engrossing desire . . . morphia. And oh! the vain, vain attempt to break this bondage, the labor worse than useless—a minnow struggling to break the toils that bind a Triton!—Anonymous

Although addiction showed a lack of moral fibre, there was no shame in taking opium; almost everyone did at some point or other, as can be seen by the many diaries, letters and novels by and about opium-eating doctors, aristocrats and, especially, writers. These documents give us an entrée into both the positive and the negative worlds of opium. We can read, for instance, in correspondence by Elizabeth Barrett Browning, who suffered from the pains of various ailments, her declaration that she took from opium "life & heart & sleep & calm." Opium was seen as a psychological boost as well; Thomas De Quincey was convinced that whereas "wine robs a man of his self-possession; opium sustains and reinforces it."[8] Opium's drawbacks, of which there were many, were commonly arrayed in confessional literature; addicts wrote of their sense of paranoia and restlessness, along with troubling physical side effects such as constipation, nausea, impotence and dependence.

But opium has an even darker aspect than its addictiveness; it's a poison and was implicated in numerous accidental and intentional deaths. This phenomenon was frequently incorporated into literature as a warning that opium abuse was a terrible side effect of poverty and disease.

Why has this drug that is at once so beneficial and so malevolent captivated those who have taken it and

La Morphine "In Paris alone, there are more than three hundred thousand scum who shoot up with morphine, drink ether, swallow hashish, smoke opium. . . ."[7]

Facing page: A woman stands over her drunken husband and says, "Ugh! It's shameful. Take morphine, it's less disgusting." Art by Forain, *Le Courrier français,* 28 June 1896.

Below: The Serpent Cigarette. Tobacco was seen by some as a more pressing problem than narcotics. *Harper's Weekly,* 14 October 1882, 651.

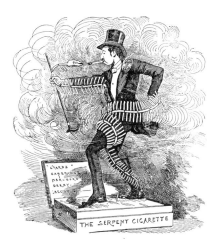

THE SERPENT CIGARETTE

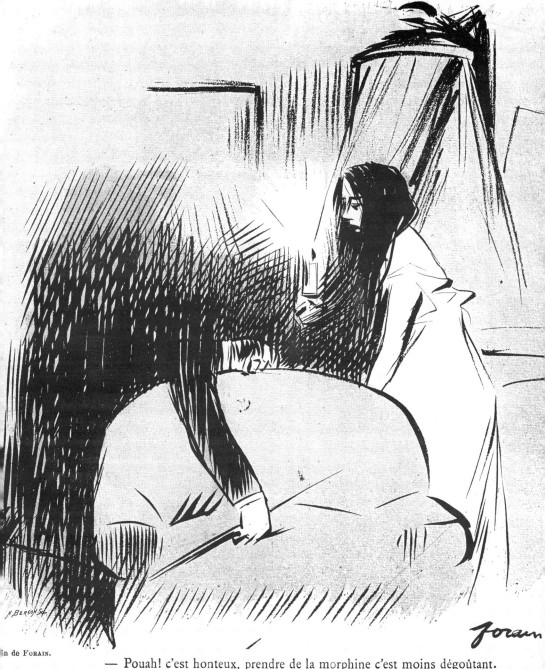

— Pouah! c'est honteux, prendre de la morphine c'est moins dégoûtant.

those who wouldn't dream of doing so? The search for the answer to this question has led me through tangled and often bizarre histories, a labyrinth of apothecary shops, laboratories, law courts, doctors' offices, nightclubs and Victorian parlours.

Essays, medical theses and newspaper reports, from as early as the 1600s, offer consistently contradictory portrayals of opium. Even De Quincey, opium's best-known promoter, couldn't decide if he was for opium or against it, so he argued on both sides. Intimate correspondence and diaries containing matter-of-fact admissions of opium dependency on the one hand or tormented confessions on the other have further clouded the picture, as have biographers loath to tarnish the memories of their subjects by mentioning a weakness for drugs. In contrast to these evasive biographies are the scandal sheet accounts that exaggerate opium's influence. Suspect statistics were spouted in incendiary pamphlets written by rabid social reformers, and even the editors of reliable newspapers lost their perspective: "1,500,000 Drug Users in America!" screamed the front page of the *New York Times* in 1923, blurring the definition of drug use to create a sensational story.

These are the words; the images, whether created by advertisers of opium products or denouncers of the opium habit, are even less honest, more manipulative. For much of the period covered in this book, images were mercenarily positive. For instance, nostrum makers produced lovely colour cards,

CRAZED GIRL'S STORY

---•---

Miss Elmino Durand Came to This City from New Orleans Expecting To Be Married.

---•---

DESERTED BY A PHYSICIAN.

---•---

Frenzied by Her Position, the Girl Took Morphine Pellets in an Effort to Die.

---•---

WANDERED TO JERSEY CITY.

---•---

Above: "Crazed Girl's Story." Sensational stories of suicide attempts by drug overdose regularly appeared in American newspapers such as the *New York Herald*, 1 May 1896, 14.

Facing page: The Needle by Sloane M. Britain. Every vice available to woman is explored in this story of once-moral Gina, whose lust knows no bounds after she becomes addicted to heroin. All of a sudden a nice girl isn't so nice anymore. Beacon, 1959.

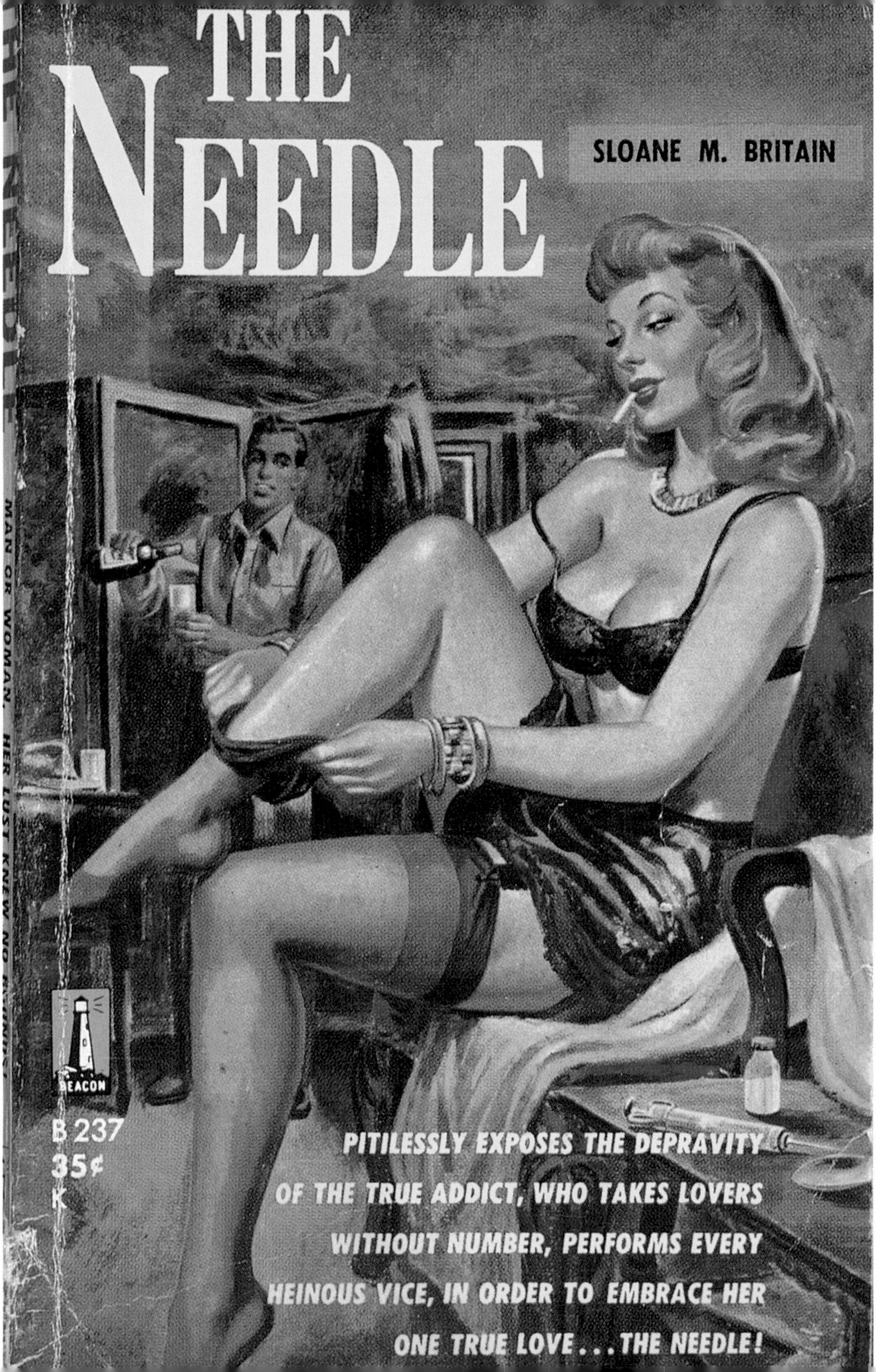
THE NEEDLE
SLOANE M. BRITAIN
MAN OR WOMAN, HER LUST KNEW NO
BEACON
B 237
35¢
K
PITILESSLY EXPOSES THE DEPRAVITY OF THE TRUE ADDICT, WHO TAKES LOVERS WITHOUT NUMBER, PERFORMS EVERY HEINOUS VICE, IN ORDER TO EMBRACE HER ONE TRUE LOVE . . . THE NEEDLE!

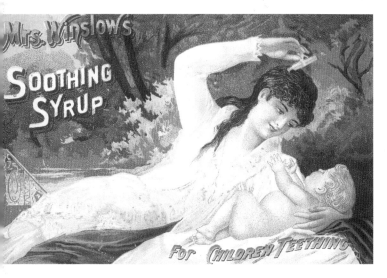

Left: 1887 Trade card for Mrs. Winslow's Soothing Syrup, a popular medicine during the 1880s and 1890s.

Facing page: Human Wreckage, US 1923, a drug exposé film produced by and starring Dorothy Davenport (pictured here, seated) in response to her husband Wallace Reid's morphine-related death. The film also starred Bessie Love (the woman shooting up in the doorway) as the suicidal addict Mary; George Clark played the role of her baby. Courtesy the Library of Congress

showing tender mothers soothing their babies with syrups made of opium and 90 proof alcohol. Up to the mid-nineteenth century, artists depicting social issues concentrated on intemperance and opium smoking. Censorious images against opium medicines appeared by the 1870s, shortly after injecting morphine became fashionable and the tragic consequences of this new practice could be assessed. By the 1910s, filmmakers were toying with drug themes, and from the '20s on books and magazines portrayed vacuous-looking drug fiends, lasciviously posed B-girl addicts, dope-crazed kids and evil smugglers.

Taken together, the written accounts and the images give us a remarkable view of our opium-soaked past. Free of the exotic and smoky cachet of the opium pipe and den, the story of medical opium is harsher, more troubling and closer to home.

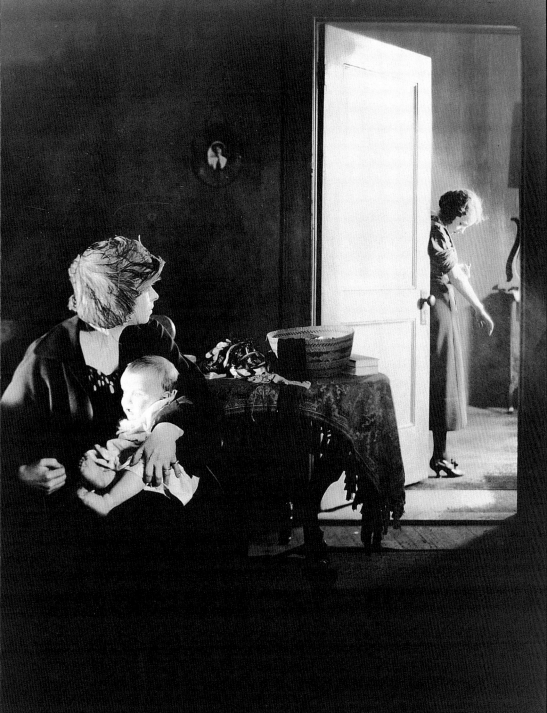

Opium at its source The opium used in laudanum and other opiated medicines discussed in the following chapters came mainly from Turkey and to a lesser extent from Persia and Egypt. Indian opium was generally slated for sale in China. From the sixteenth century on, travellers to these regions returned with lurid tales about the haggard slaves of the opium habit, fuelling the European fascination with the mysterious East. Stories by the likes of Jean Chardin, Jean-Baptiste Tavernier, John Fryer, Frederik Hasselquist, Garcia da Orta and Duarte Barbosa were widely read, so readers would have been familiar with opium's enfeebling and addictive properties. Also impossible to ignore were the newspaper reports and eyewitness accounts of the struggle in China against importing opium, especially from the 1830s on. The morality of Britain's involvement with opium became the subject of debate, both in the British parliament and on the street.

Jean Chardin's *Description of Persia* (1720) recounted mid-seventeenth-century Persian and Turkish court life and discussed opium eating as an alternative to wine. The opium was consumed in the form of a pill that ranged from the size of a pinhead to that of a pea. Chardin wrote that

> The *Persians* find that it entertains their Fancies with pleasant Visions, and a kind of Rapture; those who take it, begin to feel the Effects of it an Hour after; they grow Merry, then Swoon away with Laughing, and say, and do afterwards a thousand Extravagant Things . . . the Operation of that dangerous Drug lasts more or less, according to the Dose, but commonly it lasts four or five Hours, tho' not with the same Violence; After the Operation is over, the Body grows Cold, Pensive and Heavy, and remains in that Manner, Indolent and Drowsy, till the Pill is repeated.[10]

Opium vs. brandy

Botanist Frederik Hasselquist was a student of Linnaeus who travelled to Egypt, Palestine and Turkey from 1749 to 1752. He remarked that opium eating was less common in Turkey at that time, thanks to a decision that Islam allow brandy because it had been purified through fire, and "wherefore almost all the Turkish soldiers have, in virtue of this excellent explanation of the law, given over eating Opium, which made them stupid and trembling, taking to Brandy, which makes them mad and dropsical."[9]

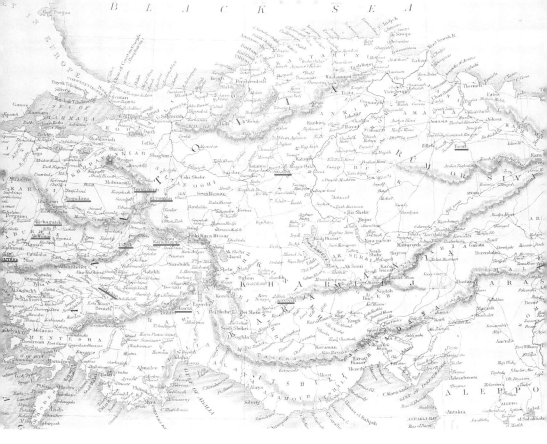

Detail of *Asia Minor,* engraved by John Rapkin from *Tallis's Illustrated Atlas,* mid-1850s.

Afyon Up until the mid-twentieth century Turkey was one of the primary suppliers of opium to European and American drug manufacturers who sought opium with as high a morphine content as possible. Several types of opium were produced in Turkey, including those from Constantinople, Macedonia and Smyrna. One of the busiest of the opium-growing regions centred on the town of Afyonkarahisar in central western Turkey.* Among the most important opium-producing towns (underlined in red on the map above) were Ushak, Akhisar, Tavshanli, Isparta, Konya, Buldan, Izmir (Smyrna), Bigadiç, Kütahya, Kirkagaç, Ankara (Angora), Malatya and Tokat.[11]

* Current spelling has been substituted. *Afyon (Afium)* is Arabic/Turkish for opium.

GEORGII WOLFF-GANGI WEDELII,

MED. DOCTORIS, PROFESSORIS PUBLICI, ET MEDICI DUCALIS SAXONICI,

OPIOLOGIA

ad mentem

Academiæ Naturæ Curioforum.

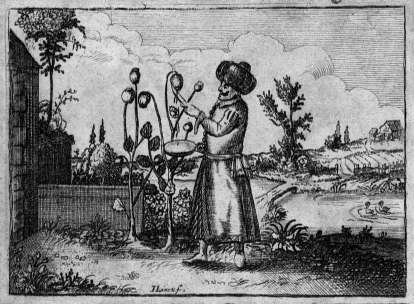

Hainck f.

JENÆ,

Sumptibus JOHANNIS BIELKII Bibliop.
Typis Viduæ Samuelis Krebsii.

ANNO M. DC. LXXXII.

The Search for Health

OPIUM'S ROLE IN THE
EVOLUTION OF MEDICINE

Answer why the drug called Opium
Doctors all prescribe as Dope-i-um.—Molière, *The Imaginary Invalid*

In 1678, satiric poet and politician Andrew Marvell sweated, then shivered while his doctor hovered over him, plotting a cure. Although a wonderful new medicine—cinchona from South America—found to be effective in treating malarial fevers, had appeared a few decades earlier, Marvell's physician wanted none of this newfangled discovery. Instead, he embarked on the treatment he inflicted on all his patients regardless of their malady. First he ordered a clyster to clear the lower bowel, followed by a bleeding to eliminate bad blood. To get rid of the food lying heavily in the poet's stomach, he made Marvell vomit by giving him an emetic. Then, in case these measures were not enough, he administered a purgative. All this was topped off by a dose of theriac, a potent opium medicine made up of some sixty ingredients. The good doctor then wrapped heavy covers around Marvell and told him to get some sleep. Instead, Marvell died.[1]

From the 1700s to the early 1900s this scene played itself out daily in sickrooms across Europe and North America. Purging, bleeding and dosing usually produced immediate, if temporary, relief—Marvell's experience notwithstanding—even though the treatments were dangerous in the long run. Opium, as a pain reliever, was especially beneficial.

The history of medical opium is the history of a quest for a surer, better means of treating disease and pain and must be

Title page of *Opiologia* (1682) by Georg Wolfgang Wedel, on the uses of opium. Wedel, who called opium a "heaven-born gift," believed that illness was caused by chemical changes in the body and recommended chemical treatments for those illnesses.
Courtesy UBC Woodward Biomedical Library.
Photo by Biomedical Communications

viewed in the larger context of the role of medicine in society. Doctors were not always the major players in this undertaking; botanists, pharmacists and scientists were more often instrumental in advances in medical treatments.

Opium's narcotic properties were first noted by Hippocrates and a number of other fifth-century B.C. Greek physicians, botanists and thinkers, but evidence that it was used medically is sparse. Poppy remedies, rather than opium ones, were recommended; one example, meconium, poppy heads soaked in water, was given by Hippocrates as a treatment for dropsy.[3]

By the first and second centuries A.D., detailed descriptions of opium as a medicine appeared in numerous Græco-Roman works. Dioscorides prescribed meconium but also referred specifically to opium, calling it the "liquor that is best, which is thick & heavy & sleepy in the smell [and] bitter in the taste."[4] Roman scholar Pliny the Elder catalogued a number of opium and poppy remedies and Galen established a system of treatment in which opium was used for its cooling properties.

One of the first true opium medicines was theriac, an omnipotent antidote compound consisting of dozens of ingredients. There were several versions, including one attributed to herbalist-king Mithridates VI Eupator, a sagacious and tyrannical polyglot. Legend has it that he had so accustomed himself to poisons as a safeguard against assassination that when he decided to do away with himself he found it well nigh impossible. Mithridate contained opium, myrrh, saffron, ginger, cinnamon and castor, along with some forty other ingredients. Nero's physician Andromachus improved upon mithridate by bringing the total to sixty-two, including opium and viper's flesh. This medicine, known as *Theriaca andromachi* (also called

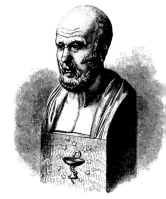

From left to right: Greek physician Hippocrates (c. 460–c. 370 B.C.), botanist Pedanius Dioscorides (1st century A.D.), physician Galen of Pergamon (A.D. 129–c. 199). All from J. Rutherford Russell, *The History and Heroes of the Art of Medicine.* London: John Murray, 1861.

Opium in Rome Pliny (A.D. c. 23–79) inventoried thirty-seven poppy remedies, including eleven specifically with *Papaver somniferum*, in his *Natural History.* These opium medicines were prescribed as eye-salves, digestive aids, pain relievers and cures for headache and gout.[2]

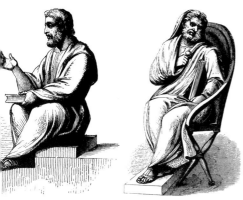

Venice treacle Our present-day word *treacle*, meaning molasses, is a corruption of *theriaca*, Latin for antidote. Venice treacle, which contained molasses, sounds mouthwatering to anyone who's eaten a treacle tart, but seventeenth-century physician Thomas Sydenham, one of the elixir's strongest supporters, wrote, "it is the most potent remedy hitherto known—distasteful as it is to many." Although it began as an antidote, theriac became a cure-all.[5]

galene) was considered especially efficacious against snakebite. Another variation, philonium, created by Philon of Tarsus, was a cure for colic and consisted of opium, saffron, henbane and honey. Large-scale production of theriac became officially regulated and was prepared in public to ensure quality. Because it contained molasses and because the most famous preparation came from Venice, theriac was also called Venice treacle.[6]

Much knowledge gained before the fall of the Roman Empire in the mid-fifth century was temporarily lost during the subsequent centuries. Although monasteries did maintain and copy many valuable manuscripts, some of the credit for our present-day awareness of ancient learning belongs to the Arabs, who kept Greek and Roman medicine alive during the so-called European Dark Ages.

The Golden Age of Islam (A.D. 800 to 1100) produced medical scholars who wrote formularies and treatises that drew from both Græco-Roman and Arab *materia medica*. One of the many opium-laced remedies listed in Arab scholar al-Kindi's work *Aqrābādhīn* was a composite of thirty-one ingredients, including frankincense, yellow sulfur, henbane and myrrh. It was guaranteed to cure insanity, epilepsy and colds. Another, for eye fatigue, consisted of opium, saffron, burnt vitriol, verdigris and hematite. In light of the henbane and vitriol, one can't help but agree with the invocation that accompanies many of the recipes: "It is useful, with God's help."[7]

At this time apothecaries who diagnosed illnesses and prescribed treatments were instrumental in bringing drugs such as

Antiquated maladies treated with opium

❧Ague (intermittent fever)

❧Cholera morbus (cholera limited to August and
September, characterized by vomiting and
the dejection of depraved humours)

❧Depuratory fever (experienced in London in
1661–64)

❧Diarrhoea frigida (liquid stools produced by
exposing the naked body to cold air)

❧Dropsy (swelling and difficulty in breathing)

❧Febris inirritativa (inirritative fever, characterized
by weak pulse and putridity)

❧Gout (intense pain, usually starting in the feet, from
overeating and heavy drinking)

❧Gripes (chills followed by fever and diarrhoea,
accompanied by great pain)

❧Hypochondriasis (men, obstruction of spleen
or gut, resulting in indigestion and flatulency)

❧Hysteralgia frigida (women, cold pain in the uterus)

❧Hysteria (women, resulting in apoplexy, epilepsy
and palsy)

❧Hysterical colic (agonizing pain in the stomach accompanied by vomiting
of green matters)

❧Iliac passion (a condition in which the action of the bowels is reversed)

❧Painter's colic (from inhaling lead)

❧Pocky itch (eruption of the skin)

❧Psora ebriorum (skin eruptions in elderly due to lifelong heavy drinking)

❧St. Vitus's dance (convulsion to which pre-adolescents are prone)

❧Urina uberior pallida (discharge of pale urine when subject is exposed
naked to cold air)[8]

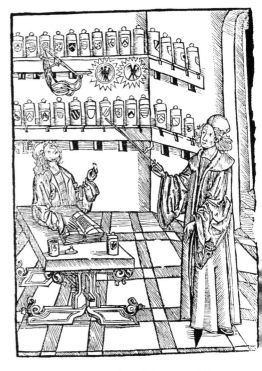

Above: The Doctor in His Laboratory.
Woodcut by Hieronymous Brunschwig
from *Hortus sanitatis,* 1496.

Facing page: Preparing Theriac.
Woodcut by Hieronymous Brunschwig
from *Destillir,* 1500.

Quacks on the Pont Neuf

In *L'Amour Médecin*, Molière refers to a theriac called *l'orviétan*, named after Italian charlatan Hieronymo Ferranti, who came to Paris from Orvieto around 1650. The Orvietan sold his remedy from the Pont Neuf:

"The gold of all the climes
    circling the Sea,
Could it ever pay for a secret
    of such importance?
My remedy cures, by its rare
    excellence
More ills than can be named
    in an entire year:
    Scabies
    Temper
    Ringworm
    Fever
    Pest
    Gout
    Pox
    Prolapse
    Measles
O great power
Of Orviétan!"[9]

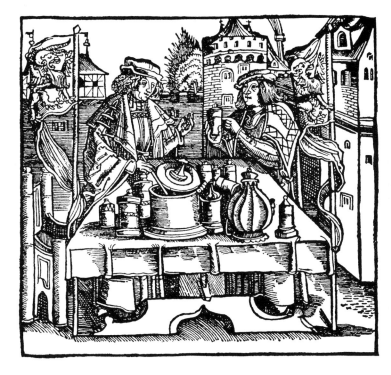

Venice and its treacle

"It was, therefore, not an ill saying, though an old one perhaps, that the government of Venice was rich and consolatory like its treacle, being compounded nicely of all the other forms—a grain of monarchy, a scruple of democracy, a drachm of oligarchy, and an ounce of aristocracy—as the *theriaca* so much esteemed is said to be a composition of the four principal drugs, but can never be got genuine except here, at the original dispensary."
—Mrs. Piozzi[10]

opium to the ordinary person. Apothecary shops existed in the Arab world by the eighth century; European apothecaries were established by the twelfth.[12] Judging from illuminated manuscripts and woodcuts, medieval apothecary shops were crammed with all manner of exotic preparations, and the old favourites—opium, mandrake, henbane and belladonna—were displayed alongside new drugs from the Americas—cinchona, jalap and tolu. The end of the Middle Ages saw the transformation of the apothecary shop into high art; gorgeously decorated majolica and faience jars became the latest accessories. The shops became dazzling venues where socializing competed with medical consultations.

The advent of printing in 1455 increased dissemination of knowledge and kick started the sciences back into life. The works of Dioscorides, Galen and others were printed and distributed across Europe, ensuring the proliferation of opium medicines. Formularies listing ingredients and quantities for a variety of medicines became standardized in what became known as *Pharmacopœia*.[13] Now doctors and apothecaries from Constantinople to Edinburgh had access to a greater number of remedies, and even more variations developed, accommodating local ingredients and traditions.

In the sixteenth century, traditional Galenical thought was attacked by maverick scholars such as Swiss-born alchemist Paracelsus. As famous for his inflammatory behaviour—he is reputed to have burned the works of Galen and Avicenna—as for his medical expertise, Paracelsus developed the theory that illness from unknown sources sprang from disruptions in the body's chemical state. His main pharmaceutical repertoire consisted of sulfur, salt and mercury, but opium also played an

Girolamo Fracastoro's diascordium Cinnamon, cassia bark, scordium, Cretan dictamon, tormentilla, bistorta, galbanum, gum, opium, styrax, acetosa, gentian, Armenian bole, terra sigillata, pepper, ginger, honey, aromatic wine and sugar of roses.[11]

Phillipus Aureolus Theophrastus
Paracelsus Bombastus of Hohenheim
(1493–c. 1541), commonly known as
Paracelsus, from Johannis Sambuci,
Portraits of Physicians, 1612. Courtesy
UBC Woodward Biomedical Library. Photo by
Biomedical Communications

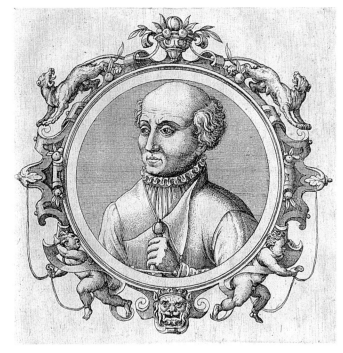

Jean Baptiste van Helmont
(1579–1644). J. Rutherford Russell,
*The History and Heroes of the Art of
Medicine.* London: John Murray, 1861.

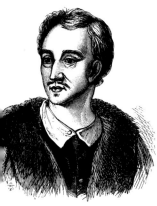

important part in his treatments. He advocated applying essences of plants and minerals, believing that they were the most effective means of treating illness, and prescribed opium and poppy for epilepsy and mania, attributing them with "wonderful power."[14]

Also in the sixteenth century, Italian syphilis specialist Girolamo Fracastoro created the complex opium medicine diascordium, and French surgeon Ambrose Paré used theriac before surgery to lessen the strain on a patient's heart. Leyden professor of medicine Jean Baptiste van Helmont, influenced by

rocation for Preventing Sea-sickness (GB 1886); Devergie's Ointment for Chilblains (US 1897); Dewee's Carminative

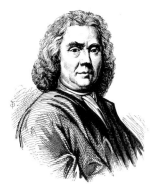 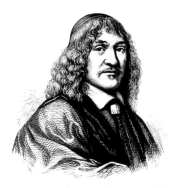

Far left: Hermann Boerhaave (1668–1738); *left:* Franz de la Boë (1614–c. 1672), also known as François or Franciscus de la Boë or de Boë or de le Boë or Franciscus Sylvius. J. Rutherford Russell, *The History and Heroes of the Art of Medicine.* London: John Murray, 1861.

Paracelsus, became a leading proponent of iatrochemistry, the theory that chemical changes in the body were responsible for illness; iatrochemists promoted opium as a calming medicine.[16]

By the seventeenth century, pharmacopœia were sprouting like mushrooms; most major European cities had their own. One of many was the *Pharmacopœia Londinensis (London Pharmacopœia)*, first published in 1618. The heavyweight opium medicines—meconium, theriac, diascordium, mithridate, philonium and diacodium—appeared in this edition, along with two truly delightful remedies: mummy *(Mumia sepulchrorum pisasphaltum)* and skull *(Cranium humanum)*.*[17]

English physician Thomas Sydenham would have consulted these pharmacopœias, and he created some remedies of his own. Although he is known for his version of laudanum, he also devised opium treatments for hysteria, epilepsy, piles, rheumatism and fevers. Sydenham was a follower of Hippocrates, as was Dutch professor of medicine Hermann Boerhaave, who attempted to create a thorough and universal system of treatment in which opium played a significant role. Franz de la Boë,

God's Hands Francis Bacon wrote extensively about opium in *The Historie of Life and Death* (1638) and claimed that the Arabs called poppy juice God's Hands. Thomas Sydenham also referred to this term, saying: "All that I know myself is that every choice and noble remedy, wherever found, receives its principal virtues from Nature. Hence, the gratitude of antiquity has well named the nobler medicines the hands of God, rather than of men. That native goodness is of more importance than artificial forms is shown by a noble pair of witnesses— opium and bark."[15]

* Mummy was thought to dissolve coagulated blood; skull to cure epilepsy.

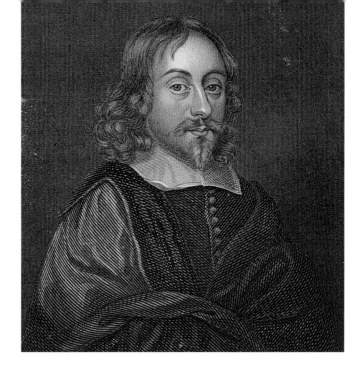

Sir Thomas Browne. Alonzo Calkins, author of *Opium and the Opium-Appetite*, wrote that Browne's "bountiful potations of whiskey . . . had been 'seasoned' from the laudanum-vial."[18] Engraving by Hinchcliff from *Sir T. Browne's Works*, vol. I: *Vulgar Errors*, 1894, frontispiece.

A Compleat History of Druggs, 1694

Pierre Pomet's study of opium's effect on the human body shows how misunderstood opium was: "Opium procures Rest, by its viscous and sulphureous Particles, which being convey'd into the Channels of the Brain, by the volatile Parts, agglutinates and fixes the Animal Spirits, in such a manner, that is stops, for some Time, their Circulation . . . so that during that Obstruction, or Tye upon the Spirits, Sleep ensues; for the Senses are . . . lock'd up by the viscous or agglutinating Property of the *Opium*."[19]

also from Holland, was, like van Helmont before him, an adherent of the iatrochemical school and made much use of opium in his work.

Opium had never been under so much scrutiny, yet it had never been so misunderstood as scholars increasingly exaggerated its powers. Furthermore, they still couldn't figure out how it affected the body and the mind or how it was absorbed into the system. It was erroneously touted as a cure for a growing array of diseases and ailments and, just as mistakenly, was thought to be an aphrodisiac because of lurid tales of venal excesses brought back by travellers who had associated so-called Eastern sensuality with opium eating. On this matter, Thomas Browne, paraphrasing Francis Bacon from half a century earlier, wrote, "Opium it self is conceived to extimulate unto venery, and for that intent is sometimes used by Turks, Persians, and most oriental Nations."

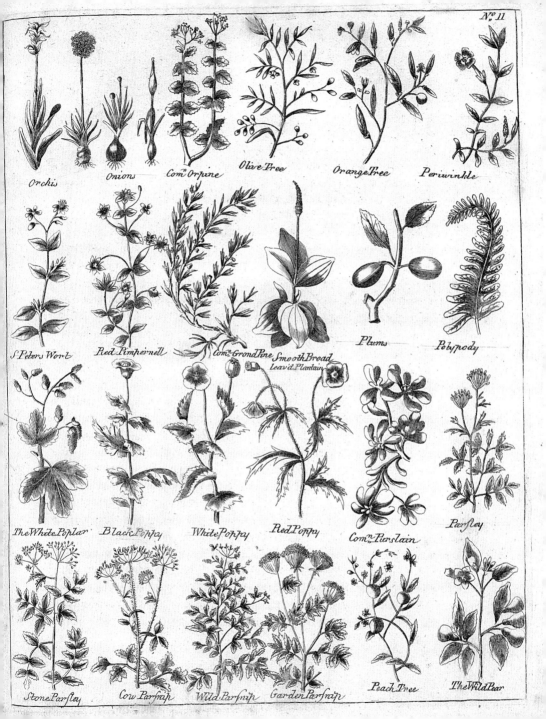

Orchis · Onions · Comⁿ Orpine · Olive Tree · Orange Tree · Periwinkle

St Peters Wort · Red Pimpernell · Comⁿ Grond Pine · Smooth Broad Leav'd Plantain · Plums · Polypody

The White Poplar · Black Poppy · White Poppy · Red Poppy · Comⁿ Purslain · Parsley

Stone Parsley · Cow Parsnip · Wild Parsnip · Garden Parsnip · Peach Tree · The Wild Pear

Poppies and other medicinal plants. Engravings from *Culpeper's English Family Physician; or, Medical Herbal*, 1792, facing p. 275. Courtesy UBC Woodward Biomedical Library. Photo by Biomedical Communications

Opium revealed? John Jones's discussion of the word *opium* illustrates his feverish pitch: "The *Latines* becoming *Masters* of the World, and of every Thing that was good and excellent; and all People observing their *Manner, Fashions, Usages, etc.* some of the *Eastern People* got the *Use* and name of *Opium* from the *Greeks* which they in Process of Time called *Afium* by changing "pi" (or *pi*) into *fi;* which is very common in all *Nations,* because the *natural Pursuit* of *Ease,* and *Pleasure,* in the Run of *Discourse,* changes the *harder,* and the *harsher sounds,* into such as are *easier,* and *sweeter,* when they are *like* in sound, as *pi* and *fi* are."[20]

It was also reputed to deaden the force of the report of a discharged gun, but Browne refuted this claim.[21]

A new school, iatromechanism, was established by scholars who looked at the body from a mechanical, rather than chemical, point of view. Following the theories of the German professor of medicine Friedrich Hoffman, iatromechanists advanced the idea that opium contained a sulfur that thinned the blood and produced sleep, relieved pain, relaxed muscles and pores and slowed the heart. Hoffman had his detractors; Ernest Stahl for one, rejected iatromechanics, claiming that the animus, or soul, dictated the health of the body and stressing that opiates were harmful.[22] Neither school was correct, but once again the controversy provoked increased investigations.

Experimentation on animals became essential to the study of opium during this century. In 1656, Christopher Wren, now better known for his design of St. Paul's Cathedral than for his medical experiments, broke new ground when he injected a dog with opium. Because of this experiment, Wren is sometimes credited with developing the hypodermic needle, though an effective syringe did not appear until three hundred years later.[23]

Medical documents had been written in Latin, the language of the educated elite, until 1649, when British herbalist, physician and astrologer Nicholas Culpeper translated the *London Pharmacopœia* into English, thus bringing opium and other medicines to those unschooled in Latin. Scholars considered his edition, known as *A Physicall Directory,* an ignominious effort, but other works in the vernacular soon appeared, one of which was *The Mysteries of Opium Reveal'd* (1700) by Dr. John Jones. This is a manic book, possibly written while Jones, who discusses his

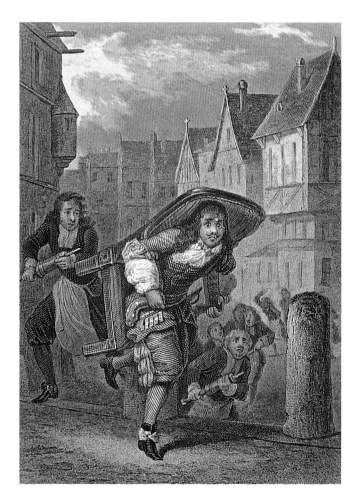

Monsieur de Pourceaugnac. Molière (1622–73) wrote about the inhumane treatment dished up by doctors in a number of his plays. Here M de Pourceaugnac is running to avoid the indignities of a clyster. Engraving from Molière, *Œuvres complète,* 1880, vol. II, 296.

The Dispensary, 1725

"This place so fit for
undisturbed Repose,
The God of Sloth for his
Asylum chose.
Upon a couch of Down in
these Abodes
Supine with folded Arms he
thoughtless nods;
Indulging Dreams his
Godhead lull to Ease,
With murmurs of soft Rills,
and whisp'ring Trees.
The Popyy [*sic*] and each
numbing Plant dispensed
Their drowsy Virtue, and
dull Indolence."
—Sir Samuel Garth[24]

Brunonianism outmoded

John Brown had much support for his theory, including that of Dr. Benjamin Rush, who practised in the United States. But one detractor, American medical student Valentine Seaman, wrote the following refutation of brunonianism in 1792: "I am conscious, that a man of fashion would not more surprise his modish brethren, in appearing without his hat crown reared four or five inches above his head, or without half a dozen buttons strung upon each sleeve, than I shall many of the faculty in not adopting the new and fashionable opinion, that opium is a direct stimulant."[25]

own and others' opium use and misuse, was in the throes of an opium experience.

Jones listed the currently available opium anodynes, including Dr. Bate's Pacifick Pill,[26] one of the first of hundreds of patent remedies about to appear on the market. And now, for the first time, medicines—some harmless, some deadly—were advertised in newspapers.

The eighteenth century saw the proliferation of unregulated remedies, yet legitimate medicines became more rigorously standardized and some dubious concoctions were dropped from various pharmacopœia. In 1756, theriac and mithridate were left out of the *Edinburgh Pharmacopœia*, though they lingered on in the French *Codex* until 1908. Nostrum making was booming, and barbaric clysters and bleedings were still common, even though scholars were carrying out scientific observations of the human body. Giambattista Morgagni, for example, conducted hundreds of dissections, looking for the means of anatomically recognizing disease. His observations provided him with a rationale for prescribing medicines, including opiates.[27]

Scottish doctor John Brown, after whom the movement brunonianism is named, determined that health was dictated by external forces; thus, opium, as a stimulant, was the best treatment for patients who were suffering from debilitating

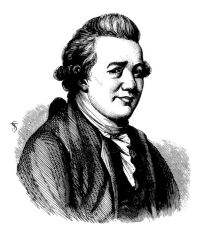

John Brown (1735–88). J. Rutherford Russell, *The History and Heroes of the Art of Medicine*. London: John Murray, 1861.

Fahrney's Teething Syrup (US 1909); Dr. Grave's Astringent Pills (GB 1886); Dr. Grinrod's Remedy for Spasms (GB 1886);

ailments. Samuel Crumpe conducted experiments, including many on himself, to support Brown's theory.[29]

Opium played a large part in the practice of English physician Erasmus Darwin, grandfather of Charles Darwin. Darwin prescribed opium for his first wife, Mary, who died in agony at the age of thirty. In 1778, Darwin gave three-year-old Milly Pole, who was losing weight and energy (and whose mother became Darwin's second wife), alarming quantities of opium. Milly recovered, presumably paving the way for a happy marriage. In 1779, Darwin tried electric shock and then opium to treat the convulsions and paralysis suffered by Josiah Wedgwood's infant daughter, Mary-Anne. Darwin reportedly said, "All the boasted nostrums only take up time . . . If they contain opium, they will often relieve; but the common ones are only *animal charcoal*."[30]

Darwin also treated Josiah's son Tom, advising him to take rhubarb and opium every night for months; Tom never recovered from the experience. Biographer King-Hele notes that "although Darwin knew of opium addiction . . . he did not realize the danger of his treatments."[31]

Darwin declined an offer to become King George III's physician. Given his penchant for prescribing opium and George's for taking it, it is unlikely that the king would have benefitted from Darwin's ministrations. Darwin was also the author of several works, including *Zoonomia* (1796), a compendium of his observations on both physical and psychological disorders in which opium is a frequently cited remedy.[32]

Most eighteenth-century doctors favoured opium, but voices of dissent could be heard. Cautionary publications included Richard Mead's *Mechanical Account of Poisons* (1702),

Kidney stones In his book *Zoonomia*, Erasmus Darwin suggested the following course of treatment for *Calculus renis*, or kidney stones: abstinence, cool dress, diluents, frequent horizontal rest, frequent change of posture, bathing of the loins every morning in cool water and venesection. If this didn't work, the patient could always try opium, first as a clyster, then orally. If that failed, Darwin recommended electric shocks through the kidney, followed by an opiate.[28]

The Apothecary. Engraved from a painting by H. S. Marks and exhibited at the Royal Academy of London in 1876. *The Graphic,* 8 July 1876.

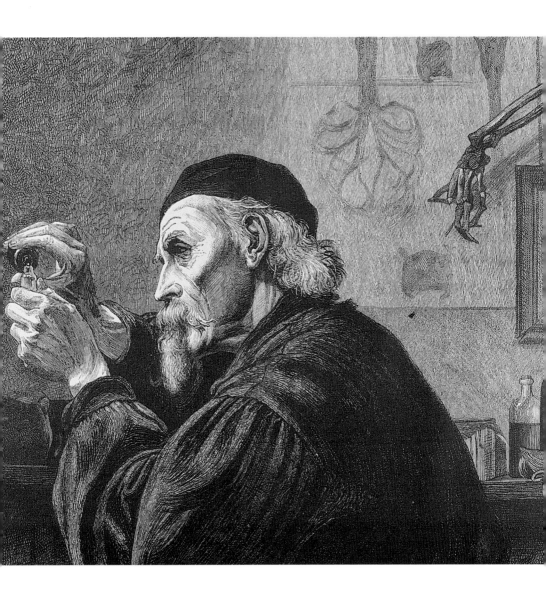

James' Soothing Syrup, with heroin (US 1909); Dr. J.C. Brown's Unequaled Liquid Drops (US 1919); Dr. J. Collis

Balthasar Ludwig Tralles's *Usus opii salubris et noxius* (c. 1757); and Robert Hamilton's *Practical Hints on Opium Considered as a Poison* (1790).

Scholars continued to subject themselves to opium; the enthusiasm evident in self-experimenter George Young's *A Treatise on Opium* (1753) was probably due to Young's own ill health; he was plagued by insomnia, bowel problems and colds. When a moderate dose of twenty drops of laudanum allayed his cough, Young tried thirty. He became drowsy and feverish, his face swelled up, his tongue turned white and his chest became constricted. When he took forty drops, he was seized with hoarseness and giddiness, his ears rang and he suffered a restless and confused sleep. Once, after throwing up some disagreeable food he had eaten, he "immediately took thirty drops of *laudanum*, which . . . made me so excessively sick, that I wished heartily for [the vomiting to] return."[33]

But sacrificial physicians couldn't be counted on for first-hand opium analyses in every instance. For one thing, they were

Thesis by Joannes-Baptista Jacquot, "Can opium cure all pain?" (An in omni dolore curando opium?), 1774. He concluded that opium was not a panacea.

A skeptic in the laboratory
George Young scoffed at the idea of injecting opium into the veins of living animals. He felt that this method would be a failure, saying "If milk injected into the veins should prove a poison, would it follow, that it must as certainly kill when taken at the mouth?"[34]

all men, so what about the women's problems for which opium was often prescribed? Young, who advised that opium not be taken at just any time, for just any reason, recommended opium to prevent morning sickness, to stimulate birth, and after the birth to ease the "grinding pains in the belly" and to reduce lying-in fevers. Young was not the only one to offer such advice; English aristocrat Lady Spencer advised her pregnant daughter Georgiana to take laudanum whenever she felt agitated. Other female complaints were also treated with opium. Young reported that not only was a sufferer who experienced an "immoderate flux" cured but her "gloomy spirits" were revived as well.[35]

After morphine was isolated in the early nineteenth century, understanding of opium advanced rapidly. Opium's active ingredient could now be analyzed as an independent substance, and dosages could be made consistent. Scientists approached their work more methodically than ever; however, they still had misconceptions about the longer-term consequences, such as dependence and increased tolerance, and believed that morphine cured disease. And still, no one knew how it worked.

The concept that opium was not only addictive but also poisonous was referred to more frequently. It is not surprising that problems associated with opium were surfacing, as opium use appeared to be more widespread than ever. Unfortunately, although we have data telling us of the increases of opium importations into Great Britain and North America, statistics for how many people used it, not to mention how many became dependent, simply do not exist. We're left to draw our own conclusions from anecdotal accounts and personal testimonials.

dial and Carminative (US 1850s); Dr. Krieder's Ague Pills (US 1902); Dr. Latham's Cough Linctus (GB 1886);

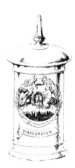

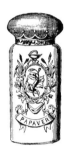

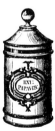

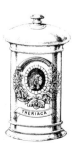

One may ask, if opiates produce euphoria or pleasure . . . then why do addicts appear to be so unhappy?—Alfred Lindesmith

If we patch together an image of a male opium addict from nineteenth-century accounts, we'll see a man of reduced circumstances who tries to maintain vestiges of gentility. He is given to spurts of fast walking and buttonholes acquaintances, rattling on at them at a mile a minute, all the while analyzing every gesture, searching for some evidence of an unspoken rebuke. Then, insulted by a misinterpreted word, he dashes off to a pharmacy, where he slyly demands laudanum and loudly denigrates the idiots who have fallen prey to its spell. Anything the druggist says is viewed with suspicion, and our man leaves the shop in a huff, swearing never to return. Back home, if he can wait that long, he gulps downs his dose. His anxieties evaporate, and he applies himself energetically to his work. Gradually he sinks into a profound but disturbed sleep, and if he's a dreamer, his dreams will be filled with incredible scenes. But when he awakens it's to a state of nervous depression. A closer look shows us his jaundiced skin and his

Left: Apothecary jars sold through the Dorvault catalogue pharmaceutique, 1877. From top to bottom: diascordium, papaver, ext. papaver and theriaca.

Facing page: A turn-of-the-century American pharmacy.

Buying opium in 1877

Meconium (Méconine) was listed in the 1877 Dorvault pharmaceutical catalogue, a bargain at 8 francs per kilogram. Morphine was listed at an exorbitant 90 centimes per gram, raw Constantinople opium for 75 francs per kilo, diacodium for 3 francs, 25 centimes per litre and theriac for 10 francs per kilo.

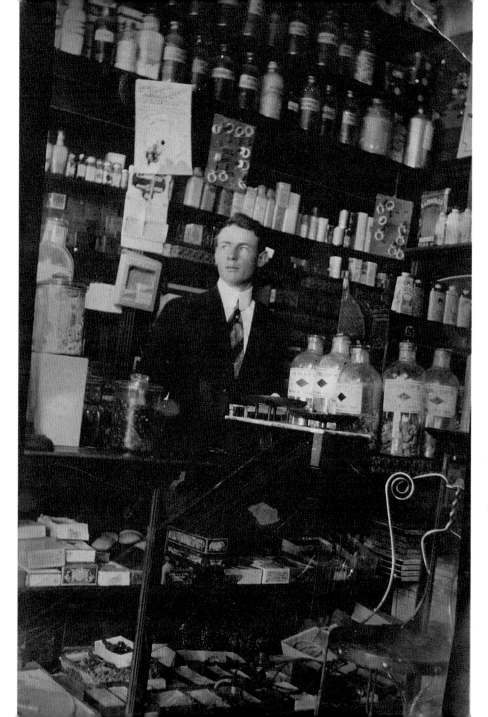

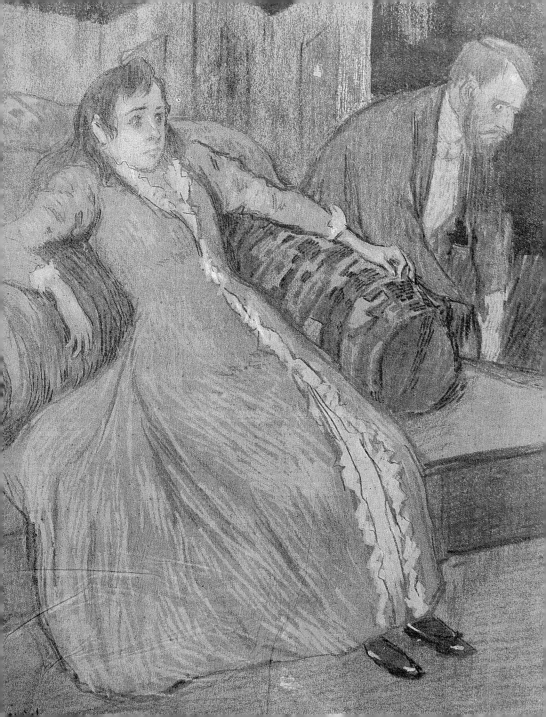

Alonzo Calkins The opium habit gave the habitué a "turbid complexion, the rugose skin, the shrunken limb, the frigid touch, the tremulous gait, even the zigzaggery of muscular movement."[36]

Les Possédés de la morphine (Possessed by Morphine). The caption that accompanied the magazine's illustration reads "They all end up in a sordid unconsciousness . . . in a state of degradation and ignorance." Illustration by Steilen for an excerpt from the book of the same name by Maurice Talmeyr. *Gil Blas illustré,* 21 February 1892, 5.

sunken eyes. His speech is thick, his lips are cracked, he's hunched over, his limbs are like sticks.

The female addict considers herself housebound, even bedridden, though she frequently makes social rounds with like-minded ladies. She openly takes her opium, and visits from her doctor are a regular event; chances are he got her started on her little habit. She cultivates a fragile appearance, writes copious letters in which she describes the symptoms of her many illnesses and commiserates with her correspondents over their own pains. If her addiction happens to be to morphine, she'll take her little syringe everywhere she goes but makes sure to cover herself well to hide the abscesses tracked across her otherwise delicate skin.

Opium use before the turn of the century has been compared with taking aspirin today. This wasn't quite the case; aspirin has never been classified as a poison, as opium was, in Britain, for example, in 1868. Under ordinary circumstances, however, there was no need to fear opium, and its benefits outweighed its drawbacks. Noteworthy, undesired effects such as dependency only manifested themselves after excessive or prolonged use.

Opium's power to addict became impossible to ignore as the nineteenth century progressed. Addiction increased in part because of the growing use of opiates, as they came to be prescribed for almost anything, including bed-wetting and ingrown toenails, for which they could have no possible benefit. Addiction was considered by some to be a disease of the middle and upper classes. American William Cobbe, a nine-year addict, wrote in 1896 that the working classes could afford neither doctors who would introduce them to the stuff nor the daily expense. He assumed that so-called brain workers, clerks and scholars who strained their thinking mechanisms, were most inclined to the habit; labourers didn't need drugs. This may have been true in the United States, where the working class was noted for its unbridled consumption of alcohol, but was far from accurate in England, where opium was a scourge of the poor. Cobbe also attributed a certain level of intelligence to the opium addict, writing that "those who are stolid, those who are commonplace, and those who are stupid have no affinity for the drug."[39]

No stars were visible in the long night of the opium habit.
——William Cobbe, *Doctor Judas*

Today we associate narcotics with crime, but they didn't always go hand in hand. Cobbe observed that the classes that furnished the largest number of addicts "were trained from childhood to abhor crime" and rarely broke the law to procure their drugs.[40] In Britain, because an opium habit was inexpensive and easy to maintain, crime was seldom an issue.

Confessing seemed to be a side effect of opium addiction. Driven by the need to admit to a lack of will, by the desire to save others from enslavement or by remorse, or perhaps seeing an economic opportunity, addicts frequently published testimonials in books and magazines. Among the volumes of abject testimonials, Thomas De Quincey's *Confessions* stands out. De Quincey, who took opium from 1804 until his death in 1859, declared that he did not write from guilt and that he wished to "emblazon the power of opium—not over bodily disease and pain, but over the grander and more shadowy world of dreams."

De Quincey Wanting to set the record straight with regard to the physical effects of opium, De Quincey wrote, "For upon all that has been hitherto written on the subject of opium . . . I have but one emphatic criticism to pronounce—Nonsense!"[37]

Géza Csáth "Opium, horrible and blessed connection of pleasure, destroys our organs and senses. The healthy appetite and the bourgeois sensation of feeling good and tired have to be sacrificed. The eyes water, the ears ring. Objects, printed words, people look faded. Sounds and words wander randomly in the tiny mechanisms of the organs of hearing."[38]

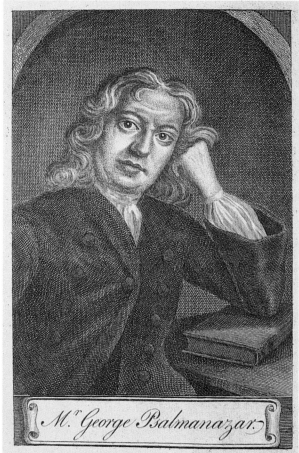

George Psalmanazar. Engraving from *Memoirs of *****, 1765, frontispiece.

It will be . . . necessary for me to give some account of that vast quantity of laudanum I have been known to take for above these forty years, and my motives for so doing, in order to undeceive such persons as may have conceived too favourable an opinion of that dangerous drug.

—George Psalmanazar

A reputed native of Formosa

Predating De Quincey's *Confessions* by some fifty-five years was George Psalmanazar's *Memoirs of *****, *Commonly known as George Psalmanazar*, a fanciful tale of how he had duped the world by pretending to come from Formosa. It was also a confession of his laudanum addiction, in which he recounted that he took laudanum to stave off a case of gout that he never had; that although he took it in large quantities, it was never so much as he claimed; and that his declaration that he'd found a way to counteract its "pernicious qualities" was false. As the lies tumble off the pages, the reader comes to realize that the whole book reads like a potent laudanum fantasy.

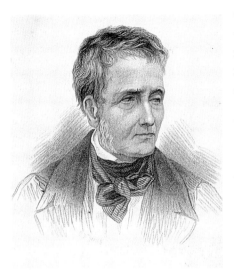

Thomas De Quincey. Engraving by W. H. Mote from *The Collected Writing of Thomas De Quincey* by David Masson, frontispiece, 1889.

The guilt that De Quincey would not acknowledge was for simple self-indulgence, not for doing something evil.[43]

De Quincey influenced William Blair, a journalist and seven-year slave to "the infernal drug," who wrote the article "An Opium-Eater in America" (1842). Blair had turned to opium hoping to restore strength lost during years of study, and though he was alarmed by the physically debilitating effects of his opium habit, it was only when the drug invaded his dreams that he'd had enough and resolved to quit.[44]

Horace Day quoted long passages from *Confessions* in his book *The Opium Habit* (1868), written to promote his program of narcotic cures. Day wrote that as he had taken enough opium "to destroy many thousand human lives . . . [he] ought to be able to say something as to the good and the evil there is in the habit."[45]

Whether good or evil, opium use in the nineteenth century was seen as a personal weakness that did not warrant the exclusion of the addict from society. This live-and-let-live attitude thrived as long as addicts were discreet but crumbled as opium's unsavoury aspects began to outweigh its benefits.

De Quincey "What was it that did in reality make me an opium-eater? That affection which finally drove me into the *habitual* use of opium, what was it? Pain was it? No, but misery. Casual over-casting of sunshine was it? No, but blank desolation. Gloom was it that might have departed? No, but settled and abiding darkness . . ."
—Thomas De Quincey[41]

The Opium Habit "It seemed as if my arteries and veins ran with boiling water instead of blood, and as the current circulated through the brain I felt as if it actually boiled up against and tossed the skull at the top of my head, as you have seen the water in a tea-kettle rattling the lid."—Anonymous[42]

Trying to live without opium

Nineteenth-century descriptions of the physical effects of opium tended to focus on the relief that opium provided rather than on the agony of overdosing or withdrawal. A notable exception was William Cobbe, who minutely examined every effect, both mental and physical, that even temporary abstention from opium had on him:

The entire surface of the body was pricked by invisible needles. If one who has felt the painful sensation of a single one will multiply that by ten million, he may dimly grasp the intensity of that form of suffering. All the muscles of the body were relaxed; there were copious watery discharges from mouth, nose, and eyes; the fingers seemed to be falling away from the hands, the hands from the wrists . . . Every joint of the body was racked with consuming fire, while intermittently from every skin-pore there issued a deluge of sweat, which speedily dried and left the skin like parchment. Above all, the soul was oppressed with disquietude, the heart fluttered like a wounded bird, and the brain faltered from irresolution. Thus tortured by bodily inquisitorial demons, crazed by wild darting nerves, and devoured by apprehension of shapeless death, I held out my hand and, placing the poisoned chalice to the crackling lips, soon subsided into physical quiet and mental torpor.[46]

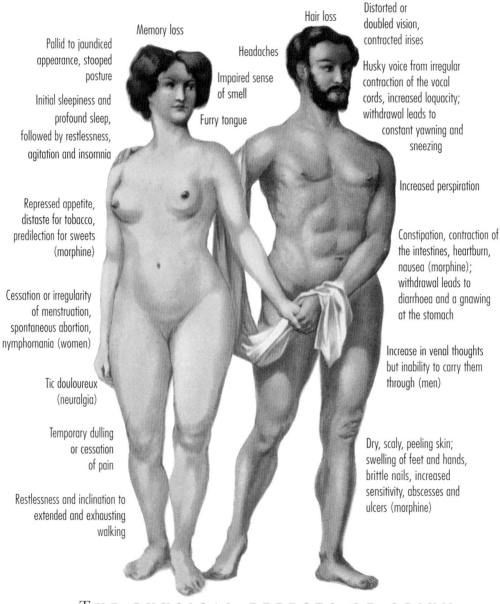

Memory loss

Pallid to jaundiced appearance, stooped posture

Initial sleepiness and profound sleep, followed by restlessness, agitation and insomnia

Repressed appetite, distaste for tobacco, predilection for sweets (morphine)

Cessation or irregularity of menstruation, spontaneous abortion, nymphomania (women)

Tic douloureux (neuralgia)

Temporary dulling or cessation of pain

Restlessness and inclination to extended and exhausting walking

Headaches

Impaired sense of smell

Furry tongue

Hair loss

Distorted or doubled vision, contracted irises

Husky voice from irregular contraction of the vocal cords, increased loquacity; withdrawal leads to constant yawning and sneezing

Increased perspiration

Constipation, contraction of the intestines, heartburn, nausea (morphine); withdrawal leads to diarrhoea and a gnawing at the stomach

Increase in venal thoughts but inability to carry them through (men)

Dry, scaly, peeling skin; swelling of feet and hands, brittle nails, increased sensitivity, abscesses and ulcers (morphine)

THE PHYSICAL EFFECTS OF OPIUM
as recorded by nineteenth-century observers

THE MENTAL EFFECTS OF OPIUM
as recorded by nineteenth-century observers

Opium and love

"Aphrodite shivers with fear
at the shadow of the poppy."
—Laurent Tailhade[47]

➤ Pleasurable sensations and exaltation, followed by depression
➤ Animation, superhuman vitality and wild mood shifts
➤ Feeling that crowds are oppressive
➤ Feeling that music is "sensual and gross"
➤ Reveries and extravagant thoughts
➤ Evaporation of cares
➤ Fanciful and fantastic or hideous and disturbing dreams
➤ Erotomania (women)
➤ Increased dosages required to appease "the insatiable appetite"
➤ Periods of energetic and intense labour
➤ Inability to finish anything, lack of concentration
➤ Willingness to stop at nothing, even crime, to procure opium
➤ Irrepressible sorrow
➤ Paranoia, easily insulted
➤ Delusions, hearing voices, seeing things
➤ Self-deception, indiscriminate lying, indignance
➤ Gloominess, aimlessness, despair, irritability
➤ Irrational fickleness
➤ Suicidal impulse
➤ Insanity
➤ Lapses in consciousness

Mann und Weib (Man and Wife).
Chromolithograph of anatomical
models. From *Album zu die Frau als
Haus-Ärztin* by Anna Fischer-
Dückelmann, 1913.

WITHDRAWAL
➤ Depression
➤ Intense suffering
➤ Aching muscles
➤ Confusion of ideas

SUCCESSFUL CURE
➤ Restoration of the senses
➤ Memory returns
➤ Appetite returns
➤ Restful sleep, free of visions

TROTRY-GIRARDIERE

PHARMACIEN

de l'École Spéciale de Paris

note de fin d'année - (suite)

Madame Perrin. 89 avenue de Versailles.

Paris le 31 Décembre 1884.

Date	Désignation	Prix		Désignation	Prix
		Report 173.20		Report	208
tembre 4	Laudanum Syd.	" 20		potion 68619	1
	Marrols	" 80	4	Marrols & Contréxéville	1
	pom. Camphrée	" 10	9	vésicatoire Camphré	1
6	Quinquina jaune pulv.	" 30	11	Vin de Coca	3
	Teint. de quing.	1 20		Valériante Pierlot	6
9	Marrols	" 80		Marrols	"
	Collyre 62949	1 20		pom. 68697	1
10	Sureau	" 10	12	Cérat	"
10	huile chloroformée	1 40	13	Collyre 62949	1
11	Marrols	" 80	16	Camphre pulv.	"
	Contréxéville	" 80		Marrols	"
14	huile d'amandes douces	" 60	17	Marrols	"
17	Marrols & Contréxéville	1 60		potion 68619	1
20	1 Valériante Pierlot	6 "	19	3 vésicat. très Camphrés	1
	Marrols	" 80		Marrols & Cérat	"
	Poudre d'amidon	" 50	21	Eau de sedlitz	1
24	Contréxéville & Marrols	1 60	27	Marrols & Contréxéville	1
	huile Cam. Camphré	1 40	29	Valériante Pierlot	6
29	Marrols & Birmenstorf	1 80	29	Liniment 68833	2
oubli 18	1 Sp. Br. Laroze	3 50		Bicarb. de Sorde pulv.	"
tobre 1	potion 68619	1 90	9bre 1	Marrols & Contréxéville	1
	huile chloroformée	1 40	3	Marrols	"
3	1 Bte vichy. M.	2 "	5	Marrols & Contréxéville	1
	farine de lin	" 40		potion et sirop 68880	2
4	huile chloroformée	1 40	oubli	vésicat & cérat	1
	huile de Ricin	" 40	8	Marrols & Contréxéville	1
	Rac. de patience	" 20			

Drink Me

Opium—opium—night after night! & some nights, during east winds, even opium wont do.—Elizabeth Barrett Browning

LAVDANVM.

℞ Opij extracti in spiritu vini vnciam vnam.
Croci similiter extracti drachmam vnam semis.
Castorei drachmam vnam.
Excipiantur tinctura semivnciæ specierum Diambræ recentium in spiritu vini facta,
Addendo Ambræ grisex & Moschi ana. grana sex.
Olei Nucis Moschatæ guttas decem.
Tum evaporatione facta ad balnei calorem tepidum fiat Massa.

Above: The original formula for the laudanum pill from the *London Pharmacopœia*, 1618, 96.

Facing page: Trotry-Girardière, Pharmacien, Paris, 1894. This receipt details a sale of Sydenham's laudanum and *vin de coca* (cocaine wine) among other medicinal items.

The opium so depended upon by Elizabeth Barrett Browning and many others of her century usually came in the form of laudanum. It reigned almighty in the pantheon of opium drugs, not only in Britain, where it was hugely popular, but on the continent and in North America as well.

Laudanum's origins are hazy. The word itself was probably used first by Paracelsus for a medicine that most likely did not contain opium. No one knows for sure, however; Paracelsus fervently protected his formulas from prying eyes. One of his students, the Basel printer Oporinus, noted that Paracelsus's laudanum reminded him of mice excrement and that with it Paracelsus "could wake up the dead." The key ingredient may have been pearl, which Paracelsus used as a sedative.[1]

Laudanum, as listed in the *London Pharmacopœia* (1618), was a pill made from opium, saffron, castor, ambergris, musk and nutmeg. Van Helmont, who lived at this time, has been credited with creating a vinegar/opium medicine called *Laudanum cydoniatum;* a similar concoction, called Lancaster or Quaker Black Drop, said to be three to four times as strong as laudanum, appeared in Britain over a century later.[2]

Who was the man who invented laudanum? I thank him from the bottom of my heart whoever he was. If all the miserable wretches in pain of body and mind, whose comforter he has been, could meet together to sing his praises, what a chorus it would be!—Lydia Gwilt, *Armadale*

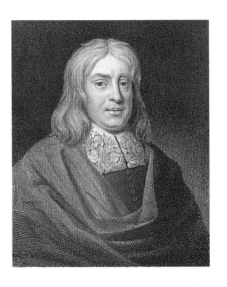

The venerated creator of laudanum was seventeenth-century physician Thomas Sydenham. A survivor of London's plague of 1664–66 (though he apparently fled the city during the worst of the epidemic), Sydenham used laudanum in many of his treatments for the disease. One of his remedies called for black cherry water, plague water, laudanum and syrup of cloves; another—opium-free—suggested lying with a live puppy on the belly.*[3]

Sydenham wrote extensively about hysteria, by definition a female complaint, and hypochondria, the male equivalent, describing them as the commonest chronic ailments of the time. Treatment involved swallowing a chalybeate (steel filings dissolved in wine), and laudanum mixed in "hysterical water" apparently helped this dreadful-sounding stuff go down. Sydenham also administered massive doses of opiates to counteract vomiting and diarrhoea but only when "suffering exceeded human patience," lest the body become used to the drug. His patients were no doubt grateful that his treatment for piles—opium and frog-spawn water—was applied externally.[4]

Above: Thomas Sydenham. Engraving by E. Scriven from a portrait at All Souls College, Oxford.

Facing page: Chemist's portable medicine chest. Owned first by William Cooper, 26 Oxford Street, then by J. G. Gould, 198 Oxford Street, London, c. 1900, this case still contains camphor, rhubarb (used for treating constipation), laudanum (shown top, left), calomel, sal volatile, Dr. Gregory's Stomachic Powder, ipecacuanha, carbonate of potash and a set of scales.

* Sydenham, in an appendix, lists this as "anti-plague water." The puppy drew fleas away from the patient, though the connection between fleas and plague had not yet been made.

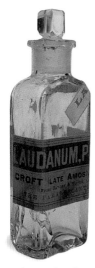
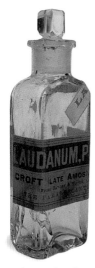

Laudanum bottles

Laudanum in the mid-1800s
was sold in glass-stoppered
bottles. The tops were covered with chamois and the
labels were often attached to a
string tied around the neck.
Such a bottle is described in
Wilkie Collins's novel *The
Moonstone* (1868) and can be
seen in Hogarth's "Marriage
à la Mode," plate VI (see
pp. vi–vii), from 1743.
Interestingly, from a chrono-
logical point of view, in *No
Name* (1862), Collins
describes a bottle on which a
"Poison" label was glued, not
a legal requirement in Britain
until 1868.[5]

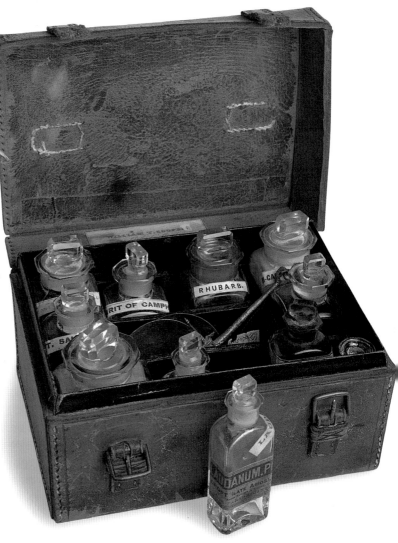

Sydenham's Laudanum was consumed on the continent in spite of competition from local preparations. In France, Laudanum Josephi Michaelis—made of opium, henbane, pearls, coral, musk, mummy and cloves—was distilled and fermented. Another distilled laudanum made with opium, alcohol and honey was created by Louis XIV's physician, the abbé Rousseau. Others followed: a laudanum by Michel consisting of opium, licorice, terebinth, camphor and saffron and Lalouette's intoxicating mix of opium, Spanish wine and eau de vie. A milder, camphorated tincture called paregoric, from the Greek *paregoricon*, meaning soothing, appeared in the 1721 *London Pharmacopœia*. Along with opium, it consisted of honey, licorice, benzoic acid, camphor, anise and alcohol.[6]

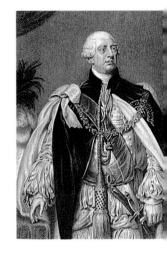

King George III. Engraving from a painting by Sir Thomas Lawrence. *National Portrait Gallery*, vol. I, 1830.

How did laudanum look, taste and smell? De Quincey referred to it as ruby coloured; Collins called it brown. Hall Caine likened it to port. Cobbe described the odour as vile; Bram Stoker, as acrid. Louisa May Alcott wrote that it tasted bitter and that you could smell it on someone's breath.[7]

In Britain, laudanum was inexpensive, readily available and prescribed regularly to royalty and workers alike. The *Illustrated London News* reported in 1858 that in the Fens district town of Holbeach "[laudanum] is sold in immense quantities, not only by our druggists, but by almost every little country shopkeeper and general dealer." The newspaper estimated that Holbeach citizens spent more than £700 a year on opiates.[8]

To understand the popularity of a medicine that eased— even if only temporarily—coughing, diarrhoea and pain, one only has to consider the living conditions at the time. In London, for example, the residents of the posh St. James Park area may have had air and space, but for most people life could

The health of the prince

In 1799, the Prince Regent had such violent attacks of pain that he reputedly took "a hundred drops of laudanum every three hours." In the same year, he relentlessly pursued a Mrs. Fitzherbert (he was an indefatigable womanizer), and according to one account, when a false rumour of her imminent death reached him, he lost his reason, took a quantity of laudanum and had himself bled.[9]

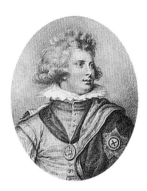

The Prince Regent (eventually George IV). Lithograph from Molloy, *Memoirs of Mary Robinson,* 1895, facing p. 162.

only be described as wretched. Thick coal smoke darkened the skies; drinking water crawled with bacteria; families were jammed into airless hovels without running water. Cholera and dysentery regularly ripped through communities, its victims often dying from debilitating diarrhoea. Working conditions were scandalous, personal hygiene negligent, eating habits atrocious and food adulterated. So, to fight the all too common ague, dropsy, consumption and rheumatism, opium was imported in huge quantities. Imports to Britain for the years 1839 to 1852 increased from 41,000 pounds to 114,000 pounds. In the United States, opium imports for 1840 were around 24,000 pounds; by 1867, 135,000 pounds; by the 1890s, over 500,000 pounds.[10]

The poor had any number of reasons to turn to opium, but what of royalty, who had every advantage yet used opium all the same? They had ample means to procure steady and unreasonable amounts of the drug, surrounded as they were by physicians who were under pressure to keep their monarchs alive and happy. The attention paid to Britain's George III and his son is a fine example of this situation. George III (1738–1820), also known as Mad King George, was given opium for rheumatism and to counter the effects of purgatives. His son, as Prince Regent and as George IV (1762–1830), suffered extensively from fever, rapid pulse, biliousness, constipation, inflammation of the lungs and "spasms on the neck of the bladder" for which he took laudanum, sometimes excessively. As king, he was constantly incapacitated by laudanum and cherry brandy. His adviser, the Duke of Wellington, despaired of ever finding him rational and watched his doctors fighting among themselves about whether or not to allow him laudanum.[11]

p (US 1897); Fahrney's Teething Syrup (US 1910); Fisher's Cough Drops (US 1880s); Ford's Balsam of Hoarhound

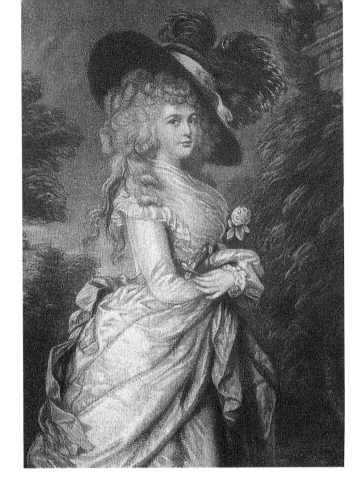

Georgiana, Duchess of Devonshire, from a painting by Thomas Gainsborough. Vere Foster, *The Two Duchesses*, London: Blackie & Son, 1898, facing p. 84.

A contemporary of George IV's, Georgiana, Duchess of Devonshire (1757–1806), was a style setter, a gambler who juggled phenomenal debts, a novelist *(The Sylph)* and a political campaigner. To counter fatigue, illness and, unbelievable as it seems, boredom, she took opium. Her mother, Lady Spencer, who had recommended that Georgiana take laudanum while pregnant, narcotized herself with the drug to cope with her husband's death.[12]

(US 1902); Ford's Laudanum (GB 1886); Fosgate's Anodyne Cordial (US 1902); Foster's Magic Remedy (US 1902); Fotherg

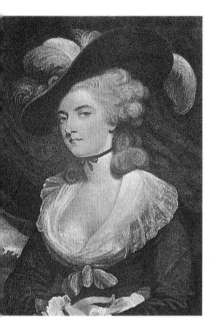

Actresses and opium

The actress Mary "Perdita" Robinson (1758–1800) was an admirer of Coleridge, a conquest of the Prince Regent and the author of the opium-influenced poem "The Maniac," which she wrote in a laudanum-inspired rush after having taken nearly eighty drops of the drug for severe rheumatism.[13]

Almost eighty years after Perdita's death, Sarah Bernhardt (1844–1923), famous for her endorsements of the coca tonic Vin Mariani, was given opium while in England for Dumas's play *L'Etrangère*. She forgot some words, causing the play to be about two hundred lines short. When she apologized to Dumas, he remarked that her omission had improved the play. In her autobiography, Bernhardt wrote: "The opium that I had

Above: Mary Robinson. Lithograph from Molloy, *Memoirs of Mary Robinson*, 1895, facing p. 175.

Right: Sarah Bernhardt, uncredited photo, c. 1903.

taken in my potion made my head rather heavy. I arrived on the stage in a semiconscious state, delighted with the applause I received. I walked along as though I were in a dream . . . My feet glided along on the carpet without any effort, and my voice sounded to me far away . . . I was in that delicious stupor that one experiences after chloroform, morphine, opium, or hasheesh."[14]

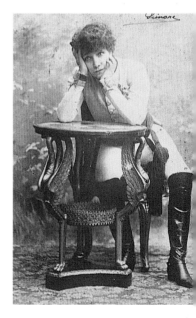

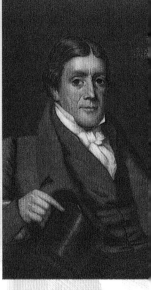

Opium and politicians Nineteenth-century politicians cannot be singled out for their flagrant use of opium, though with the pace they kept, it wouldn't be surprising if they took recourse to the drug from time to time. Lord Lytton, William Gladstone and George Washington were rumoured to be opium eaters; two politicians who had openly acknowledged habits were English abolitionist William Wilberforce (1759–1833) and American statesman John Randolph (1773–1833). When Wilberforce fell ill in 1788, stricken with diarrhoea, fever and loss of appetite, he was given opium as a matter of course by his physicians. A long-time acquaintance and fellow addict, Dean of Carlisle Isaac Milner, advised him not to be "afraid of the habit of such medicine, the habit of growling guts is infinitely worse." Wilberforce, in turn, counselled Foreign Secretary Lord Harrowby, who suffered from debilitating headaches, to take laudanum, excusing himself if he sounded like a quack. By 1821, after thirty years of regular, well-controlled opium eating, Wilberforce was in poor shape, with weak lungs, colitis and apparent morphine poisoning. It appears that even his eye drops contained opium.[15]

In his mid-forties, Randolph's neck and jaw became temporarily paralyzed, and he somehow ordered his servant to pour laudanum through his clenched teeth. Noted for replying, "dying, Sir—dying," whenever asked how he was, he was also quoted as saying, "I can take opium like a Turk, and have been in habitual use of it, in one shape or another, for some time."[16]

Most of our present-day knowledge of laudanum use comes from letters, diaries, bills of sale, novels, confessions and gossip. Although most users did not become identifiably dependent on the drug, everyone discussed here was affected in some significant way by it. Any listing of notable laudanum users reads like a literary *Who's Who*, probably because of writers' penchant for recording the minutiae of their lives rather than some inherent weakness among them, although a clergyman told Harriet Martineau "that he had reason to believe that there was no author . . . who was free from the habit of taking some pernicious stimulant."[17] Opium use was undoubtedly widespread among writers, but if the record appears skewed to their disadvantage it is likely because most nonwriters did not have their experiences immortalized in print.

On the continent alcohol was more commonly consumed than laudanum. Charles Baudelaire was unusual among French literary types in his addiction to laudanum, possibly taken initially to alleviate the effects of mercury prescribed for syphilis. Poet Jean Dorsenne, the author of *La Noire idole (The Black Idol)* (1930), declared that the French only took laudanum for illness, and besides, opium smoking was more refined.[18]

Opium's influence on creativity is a subject of unending fascination. We seem to believe that opium can unleash our hidden talents. De Quincey's laudanum-influenced Piranesi-style dreams and Coleridge's strangely haunting poem *Kubla Khan*, reputedly written in a laudanum stupor, fuel this perception. So it is with disappointment that we read reformed addict William Cobbe on the subject: "Each opium habitué is likely to be hedged in by his own wall—his fancies, doubts, fears, phantasms, and the million-and-one figments of his brain, because opium is in no sense a creator, or even a suggester of new ideas."[19]

Possible links between opium and creativity were extensively examined by Alethea Hayter in *Opium and the Romantic Imagination* (1968). After reviewing the works of De Quincey, Coleridge, Baudelaire and others, she concluded that there was "no clear pattern of opium's influence on creative writing." Those she concentrated on were already highly imaginative, a characteristic that opium may have intensified.[20]

Illnesses, real or imagined, drove most of the writers who follow to at least flirt heavily with opium if not to totally succumb to it. Before the nineteenth century, doctors probably played a major role in introducing the drug, but during the nineteenth century, for most male writers at least, the doctor was unimportant; men usually found their way to the chemists on their own, often admitting De Quincey's influence. For nineteenth-century women writers, peers were a distinct influence, as were their doctors.

My survey of writers starts on the continent with a carefree seventeenth-century wit whose opium career was launched when he contracted rheumatism as a result of dressing up as a bird. At the age of twenty-seven, French novelist and playwright Paul Scarron (1610–60), wearing nothing but feathers and honey, was chased by some pranksters and jumped into a river to hide under a bridge. He thrived thereafter on opiates, writing burlesques and satirical works and maintaining his libertine ways.[21]

Although it's not clear if Jean-Jacques Rousseau (1712–78) regularly took opium, in his *Confessions* he wrote of occasions when he sampled it, while staying with Mme de Warens, a

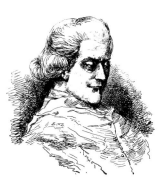

Below: The abbé Ferdinando Galiani. Uncredited line drawing from *L'Abbé F. Galiani,* vol. I, 1881, frontispiece.

Facing page: Young Rousseau watches as a friend of Mme de Warens does up her stays. Engraving by Hédouin from *The Confessions of Jean-Jacques Rousseau,* vol. I, 1904, facing p. 118.

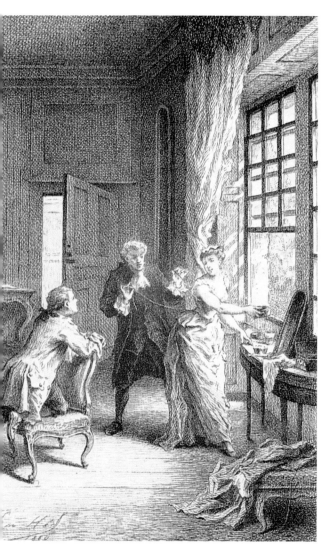

socialite and amateur apothecary. "Mamma," as Rousseau called her, beguiled the young philosopher into helping her prepare her anodynes. She would shove her opium-laced fingers in Rousseau's face and tease him into sucking them. Her lover, Claude Anet, a gifted herbalist, tried unsuccessfully to kill himself with laudanum.[22]

Another of Rousseau's acquaintances, Mme d'Épinay (1726–83), two years before her death, confided to her friend abbé Ferdinando Galiani that only manna and opium kept her going. Galiani himself had written opium into his comic opera *Il Socrate immaginario*, about a man who thinks he's Socrates but who is cured of his delusion after being given a dose of the drug.[23]

In Britain, early opium eaters included poet laureate Thomas Shadwell (1642–92), who is thought to have died of an accidental overdose; author

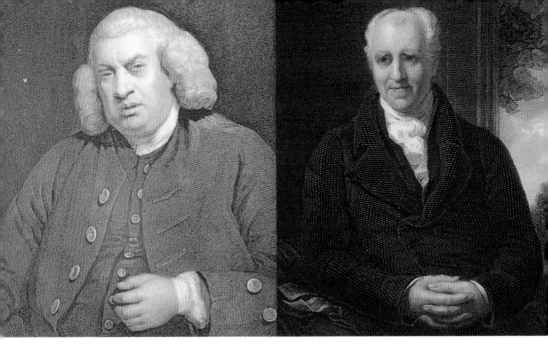

Samuel Johnson (1709–84), a reluctant opium eater during the pain-racked year before his death; and the poet Reverend George Crabbe (1754–1832), who began his lifelong opium habit at the age of thirty-five.[25]

Another, less celebrated English writer was one-time apothecary assistant Philip Thicknesse (1719–92). An opium eater from the age of twenty-three, Thicknesse was enthusiastic about the drug's rejuvenating qualities. Take it in large enough doses, he counselled, as proof citing the Countess of Desmond, who could credit opium for her 140 years on this earth. In 1749, Thicknesse and his family came down with diphtheria; only he was spared. During his illness, he stayed at a Captain Rigg's and while there tried to steal some laudanum. Thicknesse wrote that "Rigg knowing me to be an old offender in taking laudenum [sic], had cautiously locked his bottle up, lest I should be tempted to deal more freely with it than I ought."[26]

Top, left: Samuel Johnson. Engraving by W. Holl from a portrait by Sir J. Reynolds.

Top, right: George Crabbe. Engraving by E. Finden from a painting by T. Phillips. *Life and Poems of the Rev. George Crabbe,* vol. VIII, 1834, frontispiece.

Some laudanum euphemisms

"dangerous comforter"
"insidious comforter"
"quieting draught"
"drops"[24]

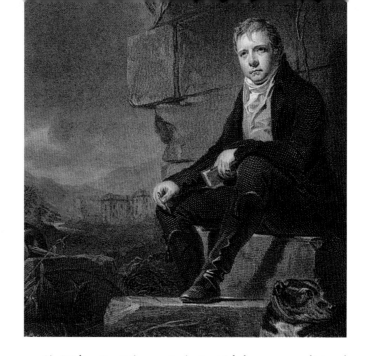

This page: Sir Walter Scott. Engraving by J. Horsburgh from an 1808 painting by Sir H. Raeburn. *Memoirs of the Life of Sir Walter Scott,* vol. I. Edinburgh: Robert Cadell, 1837, frontispiece.

Samuel Johnson "I have, indeed, by standing carelessly at an open window, got a very troublesome cough, which it has been necessary to appease by opium, in larger quantities than I like to take."[27]

Dr. Viper Philip Thicknesse, also known as Dr. Viper because of his sharp tongue, sought the company of young women for the health-giving properties of their breath.[28]

Sir Walter Scott (1771–1832), Scottish lawyer, novelist and poet, was described by biographer John Buchan as a man of extremes who led a sedentary, sleep-deprived life punctuated by physical exertion. Heavy drinking and eating provoked digestive woes, and during a dinner in 1817, he was gripped with violent cramps. His convalescence included a strict regimen of dieting, hot baths* and opium, which shrank this once beefy man to skin and bone. In 1819, he was unable to eat even simple meals without experiencing intense agony. Although consuming "liberal doses" of laudanum, he claimed he was not losing his senses and proved it by writing *The Bride of Lamermoor.* Upon recovery, however, he declared that he couldn't recall writing a word of it and, furthermore, found it "monstrous, gross and grotesque."[29]

* Scott usually sponged only his upper parts with cold water;[30] what he did with his nether parts is anyone's guess.

Coleridge and his circle Volumes have been written about Samuel Taylor Coleridge (1772–1834), who was, next to De Quincey, the most famous opium eater in history. And it's no wonder; the complexity of his addiction, the poverty to which it drove him and his family, the drain on his finances, self-confidence and productivity, his efforts to cure himself, and his lies make for a remarkable story. De Quincey called Coleridge a slave "to this potent drug not less abject than Caliban to

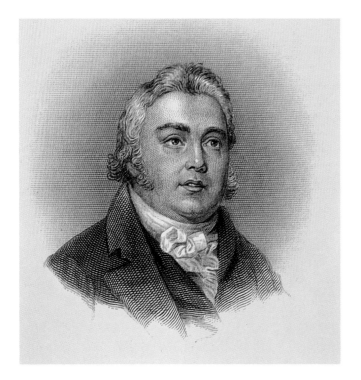

Samuel Taylor Coleridge, Grasmere, Kendal. Engraving from Coleridge's *The Friend: A Series of Essays*, London: Bell & Daldy, 1866, frontispiece.

Bhang Coleridge experimented with ether and other drugs. In 1803, he requested and received a small quantity of Indian hashish or "bang" (bhang) from naturalist Sir Joseph Banks. Coleridge then wrote to Tom Wedgwood, informing him that "we will have a fair trial of Bang. Do bring down some of the Hyoscyamine pills, and I will give a fair trial of Opium, Henbane, and Nepenthe."[31]

Coleridge's subterfuge

Joseph Cottle related a story told by Coleridge's friend Josiah Wade, who had hired a man to follow Coleridge and prevent him from buying opium: Coleridge confessed that "in passing along the quay, where the ships were moored, he noticed, by a side glance, a druggist's shop . . . and standing near the door, he looked toward the ships, and pointing to one at some distance, he said to his attendant, 'I think that's an American.' 'Oh, no, that I am sure it is not,' said the man. 'I think it is,' replied Mr. C. 'I wish you would step over and ask, and bring me the particulars.' When the man took off Coleridge ducked into the shop, had his bottle filled with laudanum, then returned to where he had been standing. When the man told him it wasn't an American ship Coleridge, of course, had lost all interest."[32]

Prospero—his detested and yet despotic master." Charles Lloyd, an occasional opium eater himself, publicly aired Coleridge's addiction in his novel *Edmund Oliver* (1798).[33]

When did Coleridge first resort to opium? Was it at the age of nineteen, when he contracted rheumatic fever, or a year later after he caught the flu? Was it in 1793, when he took opium for an abscessed tooth, or perhaps in 1796, while writing the poem *Christabel?* In 1814, he confessed to his friend Joseph Cottle (who was irked that he was the last to know) that he had been "seduced into the ACCURSED habit ignorantly" after first rubbing laudanum onto his inflamed knees and then drinking it, but he neglected to date the moment. Whenever he began, he was thoroughly dependent by 1800. His habit cost him as much as two pounds, ten shillings each week, and the quantities he drank—as much as a pint a day—are mind-boggling.[34]

Of others in his circle, Tom Wedgwood was a confirmed opium addict and poet Robert Southey a possible one. And Coleridge's associate George Burnett reportedly died at age thirty-five from his opium habit. William Wordsworth may or may not have used laudanum; his health was often poor, but his sister, Dorothy, documented her use in her diary along with an endless litany of both her and her brother's aches and pains.[35]

As the author of *The Confessions of an English Opium-Eater* (1821), essayist and critic Thomas De Quincey (1785–1859) became the self-appointed spokesman for opium addicts for an entire century. De Quincey, emotionally and physically delicate, attributed his first use of opium to a rheumatic toothache that developed after he went to bed with wet hair. He took exception to Coleridge's accusation that he had been "so notoriously charmed by fairies against pain, [that he] must have resorted to opium in the abominable character of an adventurous voluptuary."

De Quincey's consumption varied from manageable amounts to quantities that would kill anyone else; between 1804 and 1812 he took so much opium "that I might well have bathed and swum in it." Already inclined to fanciful dreaming, he was sent into raptures of delight and terror by his opium experiences.[37]

In spite of the success of *Confessions*, De Quincey was perpetually broke and constantly cadged loans from friends and publishers. Generations of addicts blamed him for their own ruin. William Cobbe wrote that "the evils of the fascinating 'Confessions . . .' have been beyond estimate and are daily luring innocents to eternal ruin."[38]

Confessions was translated into French in 1828 by French novelist and poet Alfred de Musset. Musset was a rake, a reputed opium smoker and George Sand's lover. In his translation, he left out whole passages but made up for the omissions by adding his own fanciful creations.[39]

Honoré de Balzac was sufficiently impressed by De Quincey to write the short story "L'Opium" (1830), about an opium-eating Englishman who sought a "voluptuous death, not the kind that comes slowly, in the form of a skeleton, but a modern death." Balzac also wrote of opium in *A Voyage from Paris to Java* (1832) and briefly mentioned morphine in *La Comédie du Diable*. Balzac did not take opium but reluctantly tried smoking hashish with his opium-addicted friend Eugène Sue, the author of *Atar-Gull* (1831), about an opium-smoking pirate.[40]

Insurance for opium eaters? De Quincey was miffed that life insurance companies would insure drunkards but not opium eaters on the grounds that their lives were shortened by the habit. He was refused by fourteen companies and had the last laugh when Mr. Tait, the non-opium-eating investigator hired by insurers, died from an attack of typhus in the middle of his inquiry.[36]

Balzac. Engraving by A. Ouvré, reprinted in Eugène Montfort, *Vingt-cinq ans de littérature française*, Paris: Librairie de France, vol. I, 1920, 133.

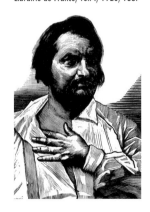

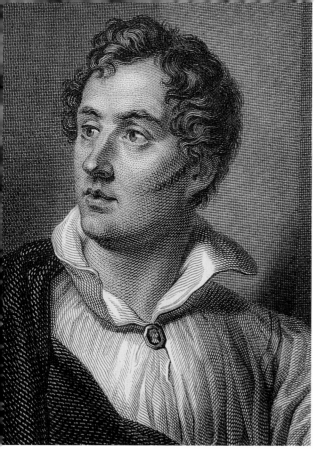

Lord Byron. Ever concerned about his health, Byron is reputed to have told his friend Lord Sligo that he wished to die of consumption, because then "the women would all say, 'See that poor Byron—how interesting he looks in dying!'"[41] Engraving by F. Sieurac from a portrait by J. T. Wedgwood. *The Works of Lord Byron*, 1828, frontispiece.

Lord Byron (1788–1824), along with fellow poets Shelley and Keats, was also associated with laudanum. A chronic dieter and hypochondriac given to extreme shifts in mood and temper, Byron apparently sought laudanum's soothing touch at least twice, both occasions pointing to a psychological desire for the drug rather than a medical need. Biographer Phyllis Grosskurth identified the first incident as occurring in 1808, after Byron received a blistering critique of his volume of poetry *Hours of Idleness*, though biographer Thomas Moore wrote only that Byron consoled himself with claret and then gave "vent to his indignation in rhyme." The second time followed closely on the breakup of his marriage in 1816. The separation was hostile; his wife, Annabella, was convinced, after finding loaded pistols among Byron's things, either that he meant to kill himself or that she was in danger. Byron's half-sister, Augusta, who was closer to Byron than is considered healthy, wrote to Annabella, telling her of finding a bottle of Black Draught* in Byron's room. She had asked Byron jokingly if it was laudanum, and he admitted it was,

* Here the picture gets cloudy; Black Draught is described in pharmaceutical histories as a laxative made from senna. Black Drop, however, was an opium medicine.

telling her, "I have plenty of Laudanum—& shall use it." Byron's attorney, Mr. Hanson, remarked that Byron had carried laudanum with him for many years. In 1821, Byron declared, in a letter to Moore, that "I don't like laudanum now as I used to."[42]

Byron's close friend, the high-strung Percy Bysshe Shelley (1792–1822), used laudanum to dramatic effect while courting his future wife, Mary Wollstonecraft Godwin. Still married to his unstable first wife, Harriet, the poet burst into Mary's family's home and thrust a bottle of laudanum at her. "Death shall unite us," he declared, brandishing a pistol that he meant to use on himself. Mary refused the laudanum, instead vowing to remain faithful to him if he calmed down. In 1814, the same year that Mary's half-sister, Fanny Godwin, died of an overdose of laudanum, Shelley left Harriet, who subsequently drowned herself. Biographer Edward Dowden wrote that just before leaving Harriet, Shelley alleviated his shattered nerves with laudanum.[43]

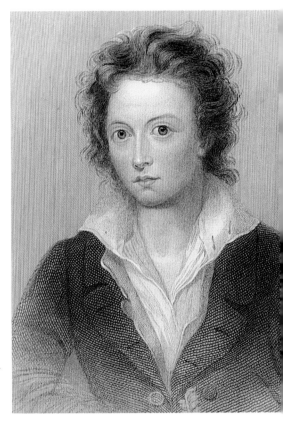

Percy Bysshe Shelley. Engraving in Dowden, *The Life of Percy Bysshe Shelley*, 1926, frontispiece.

Mary wrote laudanum into a scene in *Frankenstein* (1818), in which Frankenstein, who takes small amounts of laudanum nightly, doubles his dose, and though he sleeps soundly has terrifying dreams.[44]

To M.S.G.

"Then, Morpheus! envelop my faculties fast, / Shed o'er me your languor benign."—Byron

The Eve of St. Agnes

"Until the poppied warmth of sleep oppressed / Her soothèd limbs, and soul fatigued away."—Keats

Ode to a Nightingale

"My heart aches, and a drowsy numbness pains / My sense, as though of hemlock I had drunk, / Or emptied some dull opiate to the drains."—Keats[45]

Both Byron and Shelley died young and under tragic circumstances, but neither so young nor so dreadfully as John Keats (1795–1821). His friend Charles Armitage Brown recalled that around 1819 Keats became "reckless of health . . . taking, at times, a few drops of laudanum to keep up his spirits." When Keats became feverish and began spitting blood, his friends feared that he had contracted tuberculosis, a disease from which his brother Tom had died. TB did set in, and following his doctor's advice, Keats went to Rome. He persuaded his travelling companion, Joseph Severn, to buy him a bottle of laudanum, saying that his death might drag on for months and that it was his right to "be allowed to die speedily." His death came soon thereafter but not from the wished-for laudanum overdose; the tuberculosis had so ravaged his lungs that doctors who performed the autopsy found they'd been completely destroyed.[46]

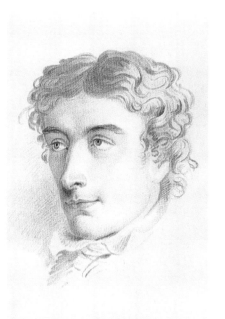

John Keats. Engraving by Charles Wass from a portrait in chalk by William Hinton. *The Poems of John Keats*, 1841, frontispiece.

Vivat opium! And may you & I live by its means!—Elizabeth Barrett Browning

Women, opium and illness

The eighteenth century produced a marked instance of invalidism, especially among women writers. This trend thrived into the nineteenth century, when a fragile constitution was not only fashionable but also convenient for avoiding the drudgery commonly associated with women's lives. Doctors, taking advantage of the female mania for ill health, loaded them down with medicines.

Charlotte Smith (1749–1806) was a poet and writer of gothic tales. She and her friend Henrietta O'Neill—both opium addicts—reportedly considered opium overdose a good way to commit suicide. In Smith's semi-autobiographical novel *Celestina* (1791), the character Sophie Elphinstone reflects on the severe shock brought about by the death of her child: "I was delirious, I know not how long, between the excess of my affliction and the opiates that were given me to deliver me awhile from the sense of my misery."[48] Smith included an opium poem (attributed to O'Neill), "Ode to the Poppy," in her novel *Desmond* (1792).

Coleridge's daughter, Sara (1802–52), an invalid from early adulthood, was frail, beautiful and much admired for her learning. In her early twenties, Sara confided to a friend that she was unable to sleep without laudanum "which I regret much, though I do not think I shall find any difficulty in leaving it off."[49] A year before her death, she wrote of being mesmerized

Conversation piece

Thackeray asked in *Vanity Fair* (1847), "About their complaints and their doctors do ladies ever tire of talking to each other?"[47]

Facing page, top: Sara Coleridge. Engraving from a portrait by Charlotte Jones, 1827. From her daughter Edith Coleridge's *Memoir and Letters of Sara Coleridge*, vol. I, 1873, frontispiece.

Facing page, bottom: Elizabeth Barrett Browning. Engraving by G. E. Perine. *Eminent Women*, Hartford, Conn.: S. M. Betts, 1868, facing p. 221.

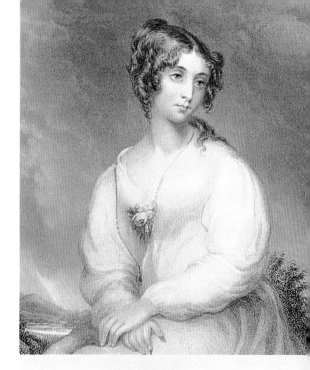

Sara Coleridge, Poppies, 1834

"The Poppies Blooming all around
My Herbert loves to see,
Some pearly white, some dark as night,
Some red as cramasie;

He loves their colours fresh and fine
As fair as fair may be,
But little does my darling know
How good they are to me.

He views their clustering petals gay
And shakes their nut-brown seeds.
But they to him are nothing more
Than other brilliant weeds;

O how should'st thou with beaming brow
With eye and cheek so bright
Know aught of that blossom's pow'r,
Or sorrows of the night!

When poor mama long restless lies
She drinks the poppy's juice;
That liquor soon can close her eyes
And slumber soft produce.

O' then my sweet my happy boy
Will thank the poppy flow'r
Which brings the sleep to dear mama
At midnight's darksome hour."[50]

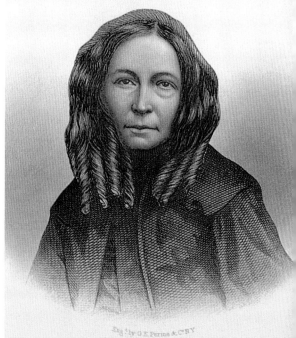

ett's Oil of Eden, with both opium and morphine

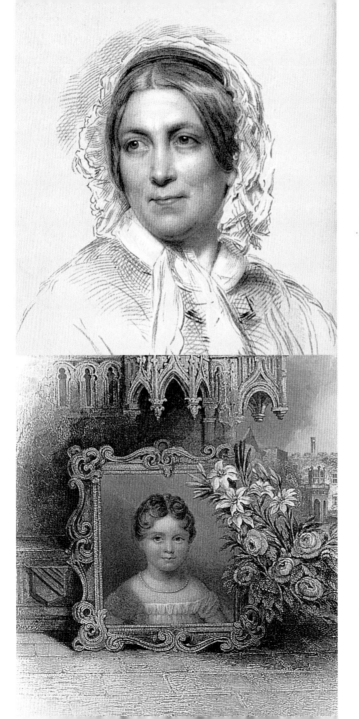

Every Man his Own Doctor, 1734

"Young Women must shake off Sloth, and make Use of their Legs, as well as their Hands. They should be cautious of taking Opiats too often, or Jesuits-Bark [quinine], except in Cases of great Necessity; nor must they long for pretty Fellows, or any other Trash, whatsoever."[51]

Top: Harriet Martineau. Engraving by G. Richmond and Francis Holl, 1850. *Harriet Martineau's Autobiography,* vol. II, 1877, frontispiece.

Bottom: Ada Byron as a child. Engraving by W. Finden and G. Howse. Moore, *The Life, Letters and Journals of Lord Byron,* 1901, facing p. 290.

(US 1916); Kennedy's Cherry Ba

by her maid. "The effect on me," she admitted, "is not strong, sophisticated as my nerves have been by morphine." And so it appears that morphine had been added to her medicine chest. In another letter, she wrote, "my medical attendant . . . now so regrets my use of morphine, himself brought me to it."[54]

Harriet Martineau (1802–76) was a celebrated essayist, abolitionist, novelist and travel writer and a professional invalid. Early in her autobiography, Martineau declared herself a stranger to opium, but later on, in a reference to a visit made by friends, wrote, "[they] spent with me such hours of the day as I could render (by opiates) fit for converse with them." During her years of illness, she became a fan of mesmerism, believing that the gimmick would provide "some release from the opiates to which I was obliged to have constant recourse."[55]

Elizabeth Barrett Browning (1806–61) took both laudanum and morphine to counteract not only chronic pain from a spinal injury and a broken blood vessel but also fainting, heart pains and erratic heartbeat. She wrote to her friend Mary Russell Mitford in 1842, enthusiastically recommending her "elixir," a potion made of morphine and ether. Her writing, especially her descriptions of the senses, was imaginative and vivid and possibly reflected the effect opium had on her.[56]

Ada Augusta, Lady Lovelace, née Byron (1815–52), born shortly before her parents, Lord Byron and Annabella, parted, became ill at the age of seven and remained in poor health for the rest of her life. Treated with laudanum, and later with morphine, Ada, following in her mother's footsteps, thrived in the world of invalidism. Her frailty, however, did not hinder her mathematical genius; she collaborated with Charles Babbage on his Analytical Engine, a sophisticated calculator that presaged the computer.[57]

Novelist Wilkie Collins (1824-89) stands alone in his pragmatic attitude towards opium, which he used whenever he required relief from arthritis, gout and, in later years, angina, neuralgia, bronchitis and nervous exhaustion. As if that weren't enough, he may also have been syphilitic. It was rumoured that he consumed enough laudanum to "kill twelve people." His pain was so intense while writing *The Moonstone* that the succession of young men to whom he dictated the story couldn't bear it and quit one after the other. Finally, a woman made of sterner stuff managed to see the book through while Collins "lay on the couch writhing and groaning." He remained addicted until his death.[58]

Wilkie Collins. Photograph by Lock and Whitfield. Winter, *Old Friends*, 1909, facing p. 216.

Collins freely recommended opium to others, though he apparently balked when novelist Hall Caine asked him if he should take it to steady his nerves. Collins also collected the names of other addicts, claiming that Lord Lytton, politician and author of *The Last Days of Pompeii*, had told him of his habit. And in his novel *No Name*, Collins paid homage to George Crabbe and dedicated the book to his doctor, Francis Carr Beard, who had started and nurtured his addiction.[59]

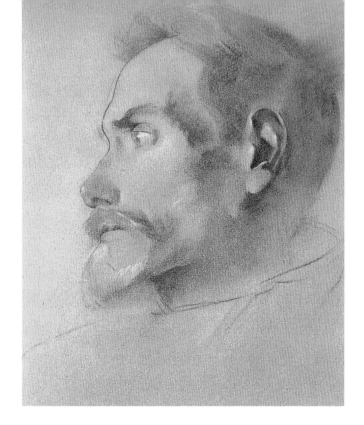

Francis Thompson. Drawing by Neville Lytton, 1907. *The Works of Francis Thompson: Poems,* vol. II. London: Burns & Oates, 1913, frontispiece.

Chatterton Francis Thompson was wise to stop and consider the fate of poor English poet Thomas Chatterton, who reputedly committed suicide in 1770 at the age of eighteen. Either convinced that he would never be successful or despondent because of a venereal disease, Chatterton took an overdose of arsenic or opium and was found "with limbs and features distorted as after convulsions: a ghastly corpse." The tragedy of his death was heightened by the arrival of a promising letter from a publisher the very next day.[60]

English poet Francis Thompson (1859–1907), an admirer of De Quincey, may have begun his dependence on laudanum at the age of twenty, following an attack of tuberculosis. Sometime in the mid-1880s, ill, desperately poor and unhappy and probably already addicted, he tried to kill himself with laudanum but claimed that a vision of long-dead poet Thomas Chatterton stopped him. He continued to live in destitution until rescued by editor Wilfrid Meynell, who saw Thompson's literary potential. Meynell sent Thompson on a long and agonizing course of withdrawal, which resulted in an unfortunately short abstinence from the drug. It was during this time that Thompson became established as a writer and a poet.[61]

Nineteenth-century literature is steeped in laudanum; its addictive hold enticed Bram Stoker, Elizabeth Gaskell, George Eliot, Stendhal, Louisa May Alcott and many others. Wilkie Collins, especially, incorporated opium into many of his novels. In *Armadale* (1866), Collins depicts the many hours a curmudgeonly Shrewsbury bookseller sits "motionless . . . in the ecstasy of his opium trance." Another character, the notorious Lydia Gwilt is beholden to her precious laudanum.[64] Colonel Herncastle and Ezra Jennings, in Collins's most famous novel, *The Moonstone* (1868), are opium eaters. Jennings, a dark and mysterious figure, conducts an opium experiment on Franklin Blake, who is believed to have stolen the Moonstone diamond while under the spell of opium.

Louisa May Alcott, herself a morphine addict, tackled opium in her short story "A Marble Woman" (1865), about Cecil, an orphan with a craving for laudanum. In this passage Cecil tells her guardian, the artist Bazil, how she began taking the drug:

> I was used to it because Mamma often had it, and at first I was very careful, but the habit grew upon me unconsciously, and became so fascinating I could not resist it. In my hurry I took too much, and was frightened afterward, for everything seemed strange . . . nothing seemed impossible to me, and it was a splendid hour; I wish it had been my last.[65]

Set in Madrid in the 1880s, the tragic Balzacian novel *Fortunata and Jacinta* (c. 1890) by Benito Pérez Galdós, features Maxi, an ugly and chronically ill apothecary's apprentice, married to the beautiful and heart-wrenchingly unhappy Fortunata. As

Armadale "'Drops,' you are a darling! If I love nothing else, I love you."—Lydia Gwilt, the maid in *Armadale*[62]

The Moonstone Extracted from the journal of Ezra Jennings:

"June 16.—Rose late, after a dreadful night; the vengeance of yesterday's opium pursuing me through a series of frightful dreams. At one time, I was whirling through empty space with the phantoms of the dead, friends and enemies together. At another, the one beloved face which I shall never see again rose at my bedside, hideously phosphorescent in the black darkness, and glared and grinned at me. A slight return of the old pain was welcome as a change. It dispelled the visions—and it was bearable because it did that."[63]

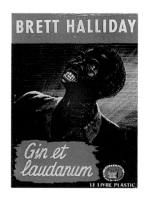

Gin et laudanum (Counterfeit Wife) by Brett Halliday. Uncredited cover art. Paris: Nicholson et Watson, 1949.

Hammett and laudanum

Laudanum did not appeal as strongly as morphine to detective writers of the 1920s to 1940s. But Dashiell Hammett wrote it into *Red Harvest* (1929), the story of a rotten town full of rotten people. And in Brett Halliday's *Counterfeit Wife* (1947), private-eye Michael Shayne runs into Gerta Ross, a well-stacked nursing home manager addicted to laudanum-laced gin.

"He was laudanumed to the scalp."—*Red Harvest*[66]

Fortunata distances herself from Maxi, his health deteriorates—he suffers from insomnia, epileptic seizures and migraines—and, like a good hypochondriac, he not only prescribes laudanum for himself, he also manipulates his whole family into fretting over his condition.[67]

Opium shows up in several of the Brontë sisters' novels, including Anne's *Tenant of Wildfell Hall* (1848) and Charlotte's *Villette* (1853). In *Villette*, heroine Lucy Stowe walks dreamily through the nighttime streets of the Belgian town of Villette after she's been given an incorrect dose of opium. Elizabeth Gaskell, who had firsthand experience of opium, congratulated Charlotte—who claimed to have never knowingly taken opium—on the veracity of the depiction. In Gaskell's own novel *Mary Barton* (1848), impoverished weavers narcotize their cares away, and John Barton spends hours in an opium haze. Gaskell also wrote of the opium addiction of Branwell Brontë (1817–48), the Brontë sisters' beloved spoiled brother, in her biography of Charlotte. In 1845, Branwell disgraced himself with a "profligate woman" who had tempted him "into the deep disgrace of deadly crime." He began taking opium and stole money to pay for the drug. Gaskell wrote, "Opium . . . made him forget for a time more effectually than drink; and, besides, it was more portable."[68]

As if vampires weren't enough, Bram Stoker addles poor Lucy Westenra's brain even further in *Dracula* (1897) by having Professor Van Helsing administer morphine to her. Then one night, after Dracula's nocturnal visits have begun, Lucy discovers her four servants lying comatose on the floor, a laudanum-laced decanter of sherry on the sideboard. She cries out: "What am I to do? . . . I am alone, save for the sleeping servants, whom some one has drugged. Alone with the dead!"[70]

We now turn to an especially tragic aspect of opium: laudanum as a common means of dying, both accidentally and intentionally. I've found no evidence that laudanum addicts were given to killing themselves, though William Cobbe declared that an addict's "suicidal impulse is very strong, at times almost irresistible." In any case, laudanum was a handy and presumably painless way to go. Alonzo Calkins studied American suicide statistics for the 1860s and determined that of 200 attempts and accidental deaths, 138 involved laudanum; of 60 successful suicides, 46 were by laudanum. In England and Wales from 1863 to 1867, he counted 682 laudanum suicides out of a total of 2097.[71]

There were countless anonymous lives lost to opium overdoses, especially in Britain. The many reports in the *Illustrated London News* include that of a young woman who was so desolate at the idea of returning to her parents that she took laudanum and died. A professor of music suffering from paranoia swallowed a large quantity of laudanum, leaving a suicide note in which he wrote that his persecutors had driven him to this state. In 1843, a man called Isaac Cohen drank laudanum and then hanged himself with his silk handkerchief, and a Mrs. Kensett died after being given laudanum instead of rhubarb. Chemists occasionally mixed up prescriptions or got dosages wrong; in 1859, a Canterbury chemist was accused of putting a substantial quantity of opium into some Black Draught. He might have escaped notice if he hadn't tried bribing a policeman.[72]

Also in Britain, artist's model and wife of poet and painter Gabriel Dante Rossetti, Elizabeth Siddall Rossetti (1834–62), was a steady laudanum drinker and died from an overdose of the

Lamartine According to Alonzo Calkins, French poet Alphonse de Lamartine (1790–1869) passed away "having survived his proper self, sunk in a dotage into which gourmanderie with opium finally conspiring had hopelessly cast him."[69]

"Sought Death in Three Ways."
New York Herald, 1 May 1896, 6.

SOUGHT DEATH IN THREE WAYS.

Made Desperate by a Lovers' Quarrel, Clara Burnham Tries Different Modes of Suicide.

FIRST SHE TOOK LAUDANUM.

Saved from This, She Used a Pistol and Then Set Fire to Her Clothing.

IN A PRECARIOUS CONDITION.

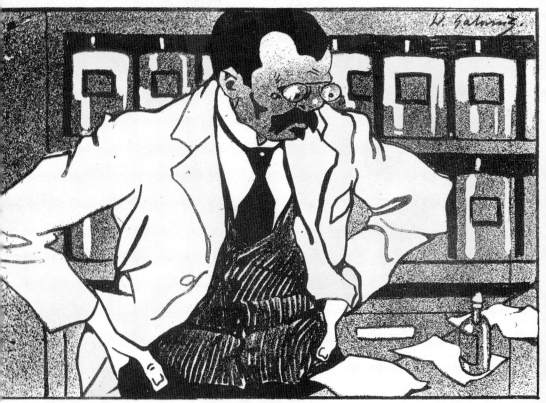

— A qui l'iodure? A qui l'arsenic? A qui le laudanum? Ma foi! Je vais les mettre par ordre *phabétique.

Les Pharmaciens. The caption reads "Who gets the iodine? Who gets the arsenic? Who gets the laudanum? Well! I'm going to put this in alphabetical order." Cartoon by Galanis, *L'Assiette au beurre,* 18 April 1903, 1814.

Antidotes to opium "An Indianapolis woman swallowed some laudanum the other day in a fit of gloom. A galvanic battery, however, defeated her plans. So, also, the Chicago gentleman who took a quantity of opium found that a couple of quarts of strong coffee which was poured down his throat was powerful enough to revive the dead. Prospective suicides should communicate these facts to friends, so that remedies and antidotes may be on hand in case of need."—*Harper's Weekly*[73]

drug. The evidence at the inquest was such that her death was declared accidental, but, given her depressed state, biographers consider her a likely suicide. Rossetti (1828–82), had used laudanum occasionally but became a chloral addict.[75]

For a country that produced relatively few references to laudanum use, France seems to have had more than its share of opium poisonings and suicides in both real life and fiction. Writer Alphonse Rabbe (1786–1830), friend of Victor Hugo, laudanum addict and author of *Album d'un pessimiste*, killed himself on New Year's Eve, 1829, with an overdose of opium. Then, eight years later, poet Hégésippe Moreau, who earned his living as a proofreader, fell into a deep depression and committed suicide with opium. He lamented that "nothing could give . . . any idea of the ennui that devours me." That Baudelaire had criticized his poetry probably did not help.[76]

Composer Hector Berlioz (1803–69), distraught by thwarted love affairs, made two "lame attempts at suicide in 1831 and 1833" by taking laudanum. In later years, suffering from gastritis, dental problems and neuralgia, he regularly consumed the drug, "which not only failed to offer him much relief but also left him feeling dazed and stupid. At least it let him sleep."[77]

French novelists made ample use of laudanum as a means of suicide or murder. George Sand's *Valentine* (1832) is about a woman who has married a boorish man whom she does not love. On her wedding night Valentine dishes herself up a double dose of opium, saying, "while I am asleep, I shall not have to think." Her true love, Bénédict, who has been hiding behind a curtain, steals over to gaze upon Valentine's slumbering face. She awakens into a kind of opium swoon and exclaims, as she throws her arms around him, "Let us both die!"[78]

Alphonse Rabbe "Death has brought its chalice to my lips; I savour the népenthès that it contains and the fatal delights of this potion. I am death's lover."[74]

Hector Berlioz. Caricature by Nadar, from *Journal pour rire*, 18 September 1852.

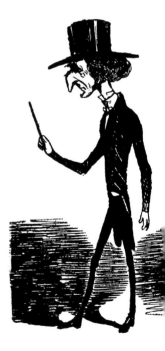

Voltaire and opium

Voltaire (1694–1778) thought he'd been poisoned when, on his death bed, his good friend Maréchal Richelieu gave him some of his own opium medicine. Voltaire reportedly gulped the potion down, his guts instantly felt as though they'd been set on fire and his stomach became paralyzed. He lived for another three weeks, all the while begging for cold water and complaining of the intense burning.[79]

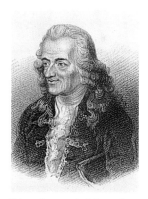

Voltaire. Engraving by E. Scriven from *Théatre choisi de Voltaire*, vol. I. Paris: Treuttel et Würtz, 1831, title page.

Alphonse Daudet, a morphine addict in his later years, included a gratuitous laudanum suicide attempt in his novel *Sapho* (1884), in which Fanny Legrand, a woman of loose morals, is jilted by her lover, the young clerk Gaussin. Friends wrestle a bottle of laudanum out of her hands as she's about to swallow a fatal dose.

Stendhal staged a laudanum poisoning in *The Charterhouse of Parma* (1839). Clélia, the lovely admirer of prisoner Fabrice del Dongo, must deal with what appears to be the attempted murder of her father, who is in charge of the prison. The perpetrator, Ludovic, a hireling of Fabrice's aunt Duchess Sanseverina (who will do anything to free Fabrice), tells Clélia not to worry, that her father's simply suffering the effects of too strong a dose of laudanum.[80]

Death-by-laudanum was adopted by British novelists. In George Eliot's *Middlemarch* (1871–72), banker Nicholas Bulstrode has been asked to watch over a dying patient, his insufferable blackmailer, Raffles. The doctor, Mr. Lydgate, unaware of the situation, instructs Bulstrode to administer several moderate doses of opium but not to give the patient any alcohol. As the hours wear on, the banker hands the watch over to the housekeeper, who feels sorry for Raffles and decides that a nip of brandy would do him good. Bulstrode, seeing a chance at freedom, hands her the keys to the liquor cupboard, effectively murdering the man. Lydgate is suspicious about Raffles's death, but he is also grateful for Bulstrode's subsequent endowments to his hospital and so does not remark on the death. A real case of a laudanum and brandy death had appeared in the *Illustrated London News* twelve years earlier. In this incident, a William Allen drank sixty drops of laudanum with three

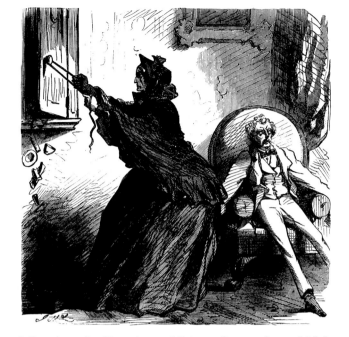

shillings' worth of brandy. He fell into a "stupor from which he never recovered."[81]

In Wilkie Collins's *No Name* (1862), Magdalene Vanstone buys laudanum and then tries to work up the nerve to swallow it: "At the first cold touch of the glass on her lips, her strong young life leapt up in her leaping blood, and fought with the whole frenzy of its loathing against the close terror of Death." Despair is vanquished by Magdalene's will to live, but rather than throw the drug away, she stores it in a cabinet, where it is later discovered by her husband, Noel, and his housekeeper, the malevolent Mrs Lecount. Lecount believes that Magdalene means to poison her husband. Collins had Vanstone and Lecount pour the laudanum out the window—and throw away the bottle as well—so that its presence would not raise the specter of murder and haunt the rest of the story.[82]

Laudanum shows up several times in Thackeray's satirical *Vanity Fair*. Here Jos Sedly speaks of crafty Becky Crawley's

Above, left: A scene from *No Name.* Mrs. Lecount is about to discover a bottle of laudanum in the medicine chest. Illustration by John McLenan, from the serialization in *Harper's Weekly,* 1 November 1862, 702. *Above,* announcements for the serial frequently appeared in *Harper's* throughout 1862.

Uncle Tom's Cabin

"Whipping and abuse are like laudanum; you have to double the dose as the sensibilities decline."—Augustine St. Clare, speaking to his sister Miss Ophelia about disciplining slaves.[83]

Hocussing Suicide and murder weren't the only crimes to be committed with laudanum: De Quincey related the story of young hoodlums who planned to rob an inn. They dosed the landlord's drink with laudanum, known at the time as hocussing, according to De Quincey, but unfortunately managed to kill or injure the other inhabitants of the house.[84]

suicide attempt: "God bless my soul! do you know that she tried to kill herself? She carries laudanum with her—I saw the bottle in her room—such a miserable little room."[85]

In Harriet Beecher Stowe's *Uncle Tom's Cabin* (1852), Cassy, a slave under the yoke of cruel plantation owner Simon Legree, bemoans the fate of her newborn child:

> I had made up my mind—yes, I had, I would never agin let a child live to grow up! I took the little fellow in my arms, when he was two weeks old, and kissed him and cried over him; and then I gave him laudanum, and held him close to my bosom while he slept to death.[86]

Laudanum use was so widespread that it would be foolhardy to try to find a universal reason that some people were able to take it on occasion without the slightest risk of addiction and others clung to it as though it were a life raft in the middle of a stormy sea. Certainly, the fashion for nurturing illness may have been responsible in part for conditioning the mind to prefer opium to alternative treatments. The ease with which it could be purchased, the acceptance of it as a panacea and the lack of alternatives were also important factors.

Although it's clear that abuse of laudanum and other opium medicines was a very real problem in the nineteenth century, the stories of habitués sneaking out to buy their "drops" pale when set against the accounts of the morphine addicts we will meet in the next chapter.

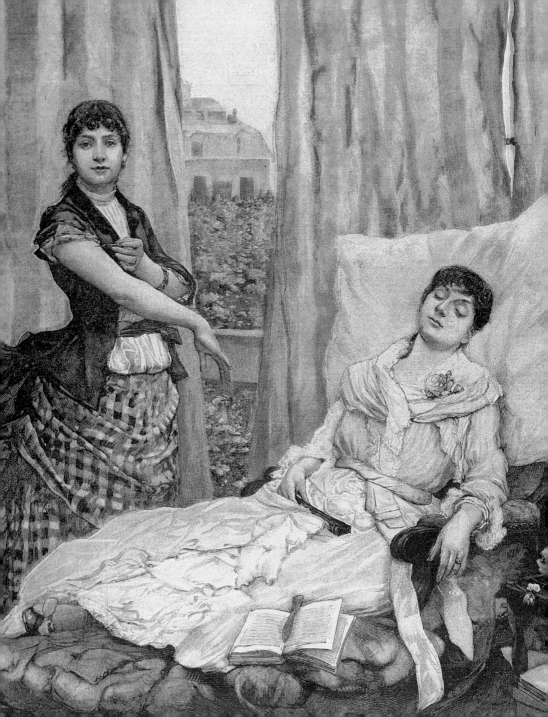

The Possessed

M O R P H I N E

Would that I could tame in me the morphinomanie.—Stanislas de Guaita, *Lettres inédites*

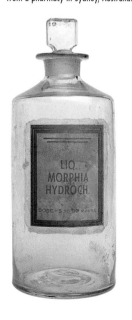

Around 1805, Friedrich Wilhelm Sertürner, a German pharmacist's assistant, somehow talked three friends into helping him with his latest chemistry experiment. He had managed to isolate a crystalline salt from opium and now he needed to see how it worked. The young men ingested huge doses of the white crystals and almost immediately experienced agonizing cramps and headaches. Sertürner quickly administered an antidote that caused them to vomit; they then fell into a profound sleep. He could have been a bit less cavalier in his approach, considering that a previous, similar trial on a dog had killed the animal. The human guinea pigs, however, survived.[1]

Sertürner named his crystals *Morphium* after Morpheus, the god of dreams. This discovery, now known as morphine, revealed the essential alkaloid in opium and launched searches for alkaloids in many other plants, including coca (cocaine). Recognition for Sertürner's work was slow in coming, but he was eventually given official acknowledgement as the discoverer of morphine. He was apparently addicted to opium and towards the end of his life became a morphine addict.[2]

Scientists had been trying to understand the nature of opium and to isolate its principal parts for centuries. To this end, Wedel, Hoffmann and Tralles, and, more currently, Antoine Baumé and Pierre Jossé, extracted from opium, salts, oils, resins

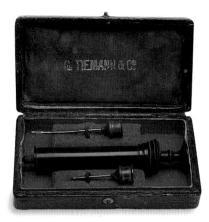

and aqueous, glutinous and vegetable matter. In 1803, French pharmacist Charles Louis Derosne had published his work on the isolation of salts from opium; his resulting crystals, now recognized as the alkaloid narcotine, were known as "sel de Derosne." In 1804, scientist Armand Séguin had also isolated a crystalline salt but did not publish his discovery until 1814.[3]

Commercial manufacture of morphine began in the 1820s in Britain and in the 1830s in the United States; in 1836, morphine appeared in the *London Pharmacopœia*. For its first thirty years, before the hypodermic needle was perfected, morphine's effectiveness was underexploited. Scientists, certain that drugs would be more powerful if they were fed into the body via the bloodstream instead of through diluting gastric juices, had been working on a method of injecting substances subcutaneously for centuries, but the means for doing so were clumsy. Christopher Wren's attempt in 1656 to use a sort of syringe to inject a solution of opium into a dog is often regarded as the first.[4]

The creation of a functional hypodermic needle is usually credited, in France, to Charles-Gabriel Pravaz, and in England, to Dr. Alexander Wood. It appears that the syringe was perfected by Pravaz in 1853 and its use refined by Wood two years later. Wood's achievement caused him nothing but grief; he apparently gave his wife morphine shots, and she eventually died from morphine addiction. Morphine injections caught on;

Left: An early hypodermic syringe, needles and case, c. 1870.

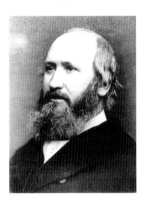

Above: Alexander Wood (1817–?) from *The Medical Profession in all Countries*, 1873. *Courtesy the National Library of Medicine*

Facing page: Carpenter's Chemical Warehouse. Advertising circular for a Philadelphia drug company, c. 1830.

CARPENTER'S CHEMICAL WAREHOUSE

PHILADELPHIA

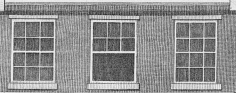

POPULAR · · · **MEDICINES**

Quinine	**Morphine.**

Quinine

Carpenter's compound fluid ext. of Sarsaparilla for extemporaneously making Lisbon diet drk.

Piperine.

Carpenter's compound fluid Ext. of Buchu, Diosma Crenata, a valuable medicine for diseases of the bladder Chronic Gonnorrhea &c.

Iodine.

Carpenter's ol. Cantharid. for producing speedy & certain vesication by simply rubbing the part.

Cornine.

Carpenter's citrated Kali for extemporaneously making the saline draught or neutral mixture

Brucine.

Veratrine, Croton oil, Oil of Copaiva, Carpenter's Chalybeate Ginger Powders, a valuable remedy in Dispepsia & Indigestion. Oil of Euphorbia, Ioduret of Mercury, Chloride of Soda, Blk. oxide of Mercury. **Prussic Acid.**

Morphine.

Carpenter's Saratoga Powders, for making Congress Spring, or Saratoga Water.

Emetine.

Carpenter's compound Syrup of Liverwort, Hepatica Triloba, a safe & valuable remedy, in hepatic and Pulmonary affections.

Hydriod. Potass.

Carpenter's precipitated Ext. of Bark, equal to Quinine, in the same doses, at ⅓ the price.

Cinchonine.

Carpenter's selection of Peruvian barks, put up in lb. & oz. sealed Packages.

Salicine.

Oil of black Pepper, oil of Cubebs, Ext. Quinine, Carpenter's compound Tonic ext. composed of Quinine, Cinchonine Piperine, Capsicine &c. a more active preparation than Quinine, in Intermittents.

Lupuline.

an extensive assortment of **Chemicals.**

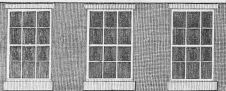

LONDON AND AMERICAN SURGICAL INSTRUMENTS, CHEMICAL AND PHILOSOPHICAL APPARATUS, CHEMICAL TESTS, ANATOMICAL PREPARATIONS &c.

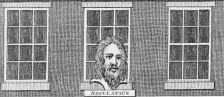

PHYSICIANS, DRUGGISTS & COUNTRY MERCHANTS, SUPPLIED WITH DRUGS, CHEMICALS, GLASSWARE, SHOP FIXTURES, &c. &c. MEDICAL STUDENTS, SUPPLIED WITH SPECIMENS OF THE MATERIA MEDICA, CHEMICAL TESTS, SURGICAL INSTRUMENTS, &c.

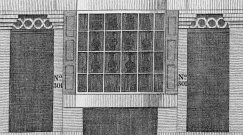

ÆSCULAPIUS

GEO. W. CARPENTER'S CHEMICAL WAREHOUSE

No. 301 · No. 301

N°. 301 Market Street the first house below the north east Corner of Market & Eighth Street

An assortment of Medical Books.

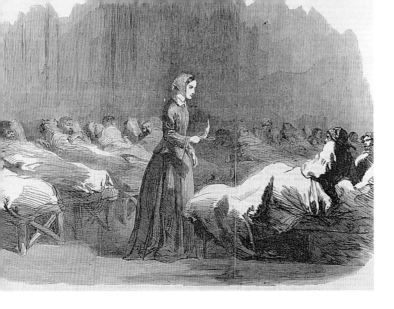

Left: *Florence Nightingale*. Miss Nightingale resorted to morphine to combat her fatigue after seeing the beneficial results on soldiers of the Crimean War. In a letter to Harriet Martineau, she wrote, "I[t] relieves one for 24 hours, but does not improve the vivacity or serenity of one's intellect."[5] In this engraving from the *Illustrated London News*, she is pictured in a hospital in Scutari, near Istanbul, 24 February 1855, 176.

Facing page: *Le Morphinomane*. The man injecting morphine into his wooden leg declares: "It's incredible! This no longer has any effect on me!" Drawing by Henry Bing, from *L'Assiette au beurre*, 27 February 1909, 777.

in 1866, a weary Florence Nightingale wrote to Harriet Martineau that nothing did her any good but "a curious new-fangled little operation of putting opium in under the skin." There is no evidence that Nightingale became addicted to the drug, though her long history of illness suggests that she had ample reason to use it regularly.[6]

Doctors were convinced that addiction to opium and morphine, which was sometimes referred to as the opium appetite, came from swallowing the drug. Injecting it, they reasoned, bypassed the digestive system and thus thwarted the craving. How wrong this assumption was soon became evident.

The hypodermic needle was a health risk in itself. It took years to figure out that the body couldn't tolerate injection after injection into the same spot, especially with needle tips blunted by frequent use. Horror stories of abscesses and infections surface in late-nineteenth-century reports. Ernest Bosc de Vèze wrote of one woman whose scars became repellent ulcers and whose arms dried out and shrank so much that she looked like a mummy.[7]

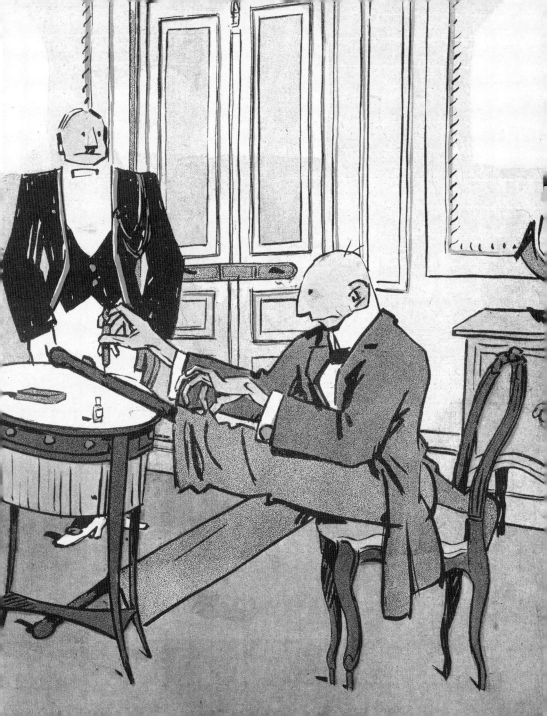

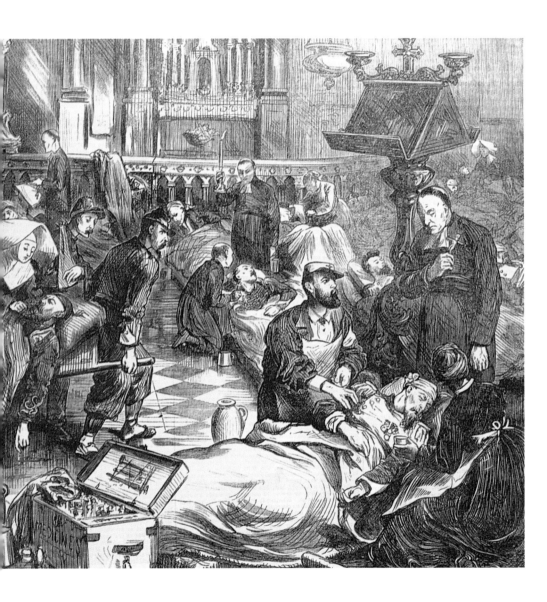

(US 1911); Moreau's Soothing Wine of Anise (US 1917); Morson's Effectual Remedies Chlorodyne (GB 1875); Moth

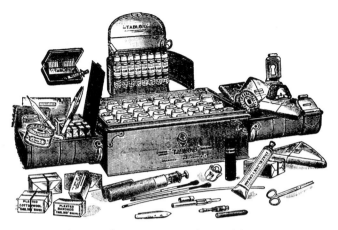

Facing page: Church at Sedan. An engraving showing the casualties at the makeshift hospital at Sedan (now in France) during the Franco-Prussian War. Morphine was heavily relied on in this war as well as in the Crimean and American Civil Wars. *Harper's Weekly*, 1 October 1870, cover.

Right: Medicine chest. Designed for expeditions, this 40-pound kit contained all the medicines an explorer would need, including morphine, chlorodyne and cocaine. Burroughs Wellcome & Co., advertisement in *Hints to Travellers*, 1906.

Louis Faucher "I began to experience the euphoria of morphine. It made the night sweet for me; I can scarcely express in any other way the subtle pleasure that I experienced. . . . Things that had seemed difficult now seemed easy. . . . It was nothing. It was scarcely noticeable. But it was good."[8]

Most nineteenth-century morphine addicts were initially given the drug for medical reasons, and it was indispensable in the Civil, Crimean and Franco-Prussian Wars. Away from the battlefields, however, in the sickrooms of middle-class homes, it was prescribed as an analgesic and as a cure for rheumatism, headaches, women's complaints and a variety of other ills. In the accounts of those who attempted to live with morphine, a desperation emerges from behind the initial pleasure, something not sensed as often among laudanum users.

If laudanum could be considered a British phenomenon, then morphine belonged to France. There, writers such as Guy de Maupassant, Laurent Tailhade, Jean Lorrain and Stanislas de Guaita were the inheritors of a tradition of drug experimentation established in the 1840s by the Club des Haschichins, of which Charles Baudelaire and Théophile Gautier were notable members. Morphine use was by no means limited to this group; however, the lives of the prostitutes, sailors and drifters who increasingly fell under morphine's spell as the nineteenth century wore on were largely undocumented.

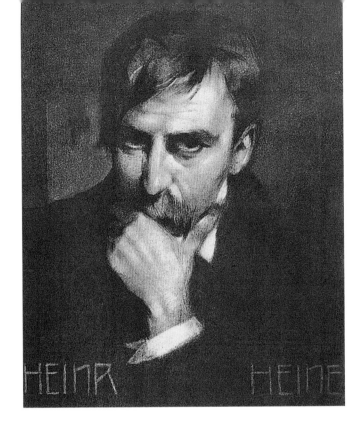

One of the earliest cases of morphine addiction is that of German poet and travel writer Heinrich Heine (1797–1856). Heine lived in France for much of his adult life and from his mid-thirties on was racked by headaches, cramps and intermittent paralysis. Treatment consisted of taking morphine and having opium rubbed into sores that were kept open for that purpose. For the twelve years leading up to his death, Heine was virtually immobilized, yet he created some of his most memorable work during that time. In his poem "Morphine," Heine writes of being held in the loving arms of the drug and of how the wreath of poppies "Upon his head brushed over my own forehead / And, strangely fragrant, banished all the pain."[10]

À la morphine

"Ah! Pierce me one hundred
  times with your needle fine
And I will thank you one
  hundred times, *Sainte Morphine,*
You who Aesculapius has
  made a God."
—Jules Verne[9]

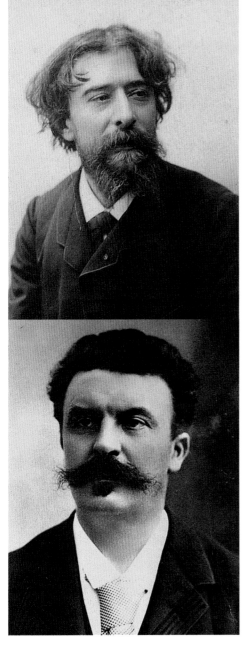

In his later years, novelist Alphonse Daudet (1840–97) lived in a rest home at Lamalou-les-Bains, where morphine flowed "like Vichy water" and "the shots of euphoric poison were as numerous . . . as those of mosquitoes." His son Léon recounted a conversation between his father and another patient, who competed to see who took the most morphine: " 'Madame, I take a gram a day.' 'Oh! That's scarcely anything. Me, I take a gram and a half.' "[11]

Novelist Guy de Maupassant (1850–93) was prone to seizures and migraines. Much of the ill health that plagued him through his adult years could be blamed on syphilis, against which he tried ether, hashish, cocaine and morphine. Maupassant was obsessed by the subject of madness and wrote about it frequently; several of his stories, including "Un Fou" (1885) and the autobiographical *Sur l'eau* (1888) are penetrating observations of a descent into madness. Scholars suggest that his insanity, though not caused by drugs, was certainly exacerbated by them.[12]

The drug taking of novelist and journalist Jean Lorrain (1855–1906) has been compared with that of Baudelaire and Cocteau. Biographer Philippe Jullian wrote that Lorrain thought of himself as "the ambassador of Sodom to Tout-Paris" and his novels, such as the wickedly corrupt tale *Monsieur de Phocas*, reflected that. From his twenty-fifth year Lorrain was in poor health and, with his startlingly made-up eyes and gilded hair, cultivated a feverish look. In 1885, tuberculosis set in; a year later, he wrote, "I have the sweet and pardoning soul of people who must die: these nervous accidents, these atrocious sufferings, these injections of morphine." He died, dreadfully, of a ruptured intestine.[14]

Stanislas de Guaita (1861–97), occultist, author and morphinomaniac, was chronically ill, possibly a hypochondric, and would lace his correspondence with remedies for his friends' maladies. Poet and critic Laurent Tailhade, also a morphine addict, commented that Guaita, "in his glory days of morphinomania," would purchase the drug by the kilo. His death has been attributed to morphine.[15]

Edouard Dubus (1864–95), cofounder of the *Mercure de France*, was a poet, alcoholic and morphinomane and, like Guaita, died of a morphine overdose. According to Pascal Pia, "his body was discovered in a *chalet de nécessité*, place Maubert. In his pocket was a Pravaz syringe. One will never know if he had purposely chosen to finish his life in such a place."[16]

For someone who abstained from drugs, the writer Colette managed to surround herself with a rather illustrious group of morphine addicts, including her lover Missy (Mathilde de Morny), whose behaviour was audacious even for the heady

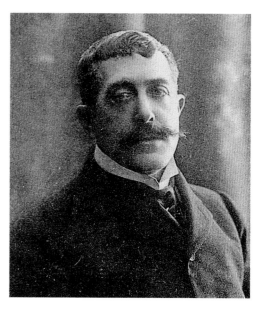

Jean Lorrain. Photograph by Boissonnas, n.d.

Cocteau on morphine

"A morphine addict's blood shows no trace of morphine. It is tempting to imagine the day when doctors will discover the hiding places of morphine and will lure it out by using some substance to which it is partial, like a snake with a bowl of milk."[13]

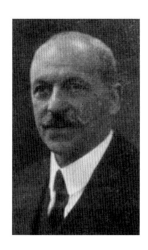

Marcel Schwob. Schwob and Jean Lorrain were close friends. According to Jullian, "A taste for ether . . . brought them together, plus Schwob gave in to opium; both had much to forget."[17] Photo by Manuel.

Jules Lemaître on the poet Stéphane Mallarmé
"He is like a rose injected with morphine."[18]

times of fin de siècle France; she flaunted her men's attire, reputedly had a "stable" of lovers and became a morphine addict. Another female acquaintance, writer Renée Vivien (1877–1909), was one of the infamous troupe of literary Paris lesbians and was noted for her dependence upon ether, morphine and alcohol. Biographer Paul Lorenz, however, barely mentions drugs, though he refers to Vivien's attempt at suicide by laudanum.[19]

Colette's addicted male friends included Marcel Schwob (1867–1905), critic, translator and author of *Les Portes de l'opium* (1891), who suffered from chronic poor health and became addicted, first to opium, then to morphine. Novelist Pierre Louÿs (1870–1925), author of the erotic novel *Aphrodite* (1896), smoked a phenomenal number of cigarettes in spite of a bronchial condition, drank quarts of the coca tonic Vin Mariani and, in the last years of his rather short life, took morphine. In his introduction to Claude Farrère's *Fumée d'opium* (1904), he wrote that Farrère had never smoked opium. Farrère, in turn, claimed that Louÿs had "a horror of all drugs."[20]

The years Marcel Proust (1871–1922) spent holed up in a cork-lined room are the stuff of legend. Proust suffered from hay fever, asthma, insomnia, indigestion and a strong attachment to his mother. His doctor told him to lay off of alcohol and morphine and instead take Veronal, bathe in cold water and stay in bed. Around 1904, he wrote his mother, asking her to buy him some heroin, though he was "absolutely determined not to take any." Whether or not he did, Proust became addicted to Veronal and Trional; he also used an opiated anti-asthmatic and, in 1921, came close to overdosing on a drug mixture that contained opium.[21]

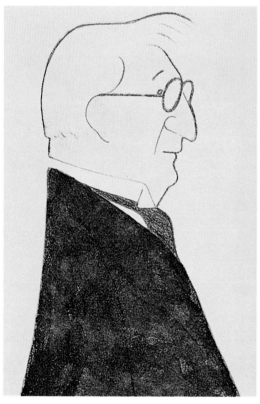

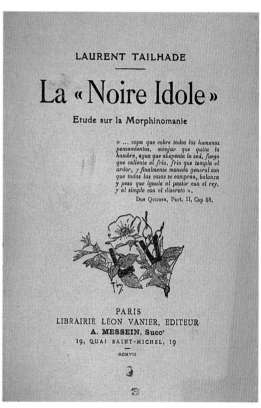

Above: Laurent Tailhade, critic and author of *La « Noire idole »* (right). Portrait by Sacha Guitry, from *Les « Commérges » de Tybalt,* 1914, frontispiece.

Setting the record straight Poet, satirist and critic Laurent Tailhade (1854–1919) wrote *La « Noire idole »* (1907), in which he tried to give a rational description of morphine and to rectify errors in Maurice Talmeyr's *Les Possédés de la morphine,* a scathing look at morphine addiction in France. Tailhade himself became addicted to morphine at the age of forty after losing an eye to a bomb planted, according to one report, by an anarchist, according to another, by a thwarted lover.[22]

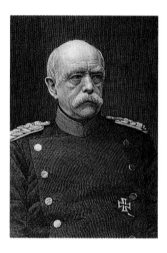

Right: Bismarck (1815–98), as reported by Tailhade, would not speak at the Reichstag until he had injected himself with morphine.[23] From Charles Lowe, *Prince Bismarck: An Historical Biography,* vol. I. London: Cassell, 1887, frontispiece.

Below: La Noire idole, Jean Dorsenne. Mostly concerned with opium smoking, Dorsenne pointed out that though the title of his book was the same as Tailhade's, his use of the phrase "The Black Idol" was more correct. Cover art by Jean A. Mercier, 1930.

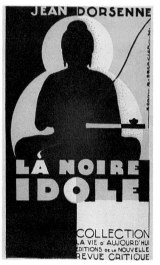

On top of the well-documented cases of morphine addiction, there are boundless rumours and incomplete stories. Snippets of innuendo creep from the pages of Laurent Tailhade's celebration of morphine, *La Noire idole.* He wrote of the morphine habit of French actor Jacques Damala, and his claim that Prince Otto Eduard Leopold von Bismarck was a morphinomaniac was seconded by Léon Daudet. French naval officer and writer Claude Farrère smoked opium, but his morphine use is considered certain by several observers, including biographer Quella-Villéger. Of French writer Ernest Renan, Jules Lemaître declared, "He lets in the saints of lust, morphine and alcohol. And with that he's happy!" Recent biographies of Colette have highlighted the alleged addictions of Spanish painter José Maria Sert, actor Edouard de Max and the fast-living Kessel brothers: actor Lazare, editor Georges and journalist Joseph.[24]

"Goodbye cares, goodbye pain! The brutal nirvana is at hand. All it takes is a little flacon containing a solution of morphine and one of Pravaƶ's syringes."

—Jean Dorsenne, *La Noire idole*

Women & morphine

We saw in the previous chapter the laudanum and morphine addictions of Elizabeth Barrett Browning, Sara Coleridge and Ada Byron. Louisa May Alcott and Alice James also took laudanum and, more notably, morphine. Alcott (1832–88), the author of *Little Women*, was given morphine in 1862, probably to combat the effects of mercury, prescribed in the form of calomel, which she was given after contracting pneumonia while nursing Civil War soldiers. Ill for much of her adult life, Alcott suffered from dyspepsia, insomnia, catarrh, coughing, lack of appetite, an ulcerated throat and loss of voice.[26]

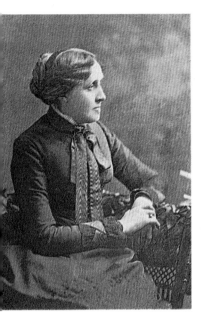

Louisa May Alcott, photographed in 1887 by A. W. Elson. Ednah Cheney, *Louisa May Alcott.* Boston: Roberts Brothers, 1890, frontispiece.

Alice James (1848-92), invalid sister of the novelist Henry James, having suffered a series of nervous breakdowns, not only took opium and morphine but also tried electric shock, hypnosis and two mysterious cures, "motorpathy" and the "Monro treatment." One of her brothers, William, had been given morphine almost constantly to alleviate his suffering before his death at a young age.[27]

Alice James

"The treacherous fiend Morphia, which while murdering pain destroys sleep and opens the door to all hideous nervous distresses, disclosed its iniquities to us and I touched bottom more nearly than ever before."[25]

*She's become . . . How do you say? . . . A morphine addict. . . .
There's a whole society like that . . . When they get together, each of
these women, carrying their little silver cases with the needle, the
poison . . . and wham! in the arm, in the leg . . . It doesn't make you
sleep . . . but one feels good.*—Alphonse Daudet, *L'Évangeliste*

Alcott's and James's morphine use can be seen as part of the pre-1850s illness cult experienced by middle-class women. As the
century wore on though, and the syringe became accepted, morphine was adopted by another, far less definable group. Bored or
restless women from all economic levels began injecting morphine, sometimes for medical reasons, sometimes in search of
euphoria. And their habit was no longer confined to stuffy sickrooms; it was out in the open, even flaunted. Reliable statistics
are difficult to come by, but numerous references imply that
morphine syringes among the theatre crowd were as common as
cigarettes. Either use of morphine by women reached epidemic
levels in the late nineteenth century or newspaper reporters and
novelists blew it out of proportion.

The wild and heady life of American socialite Evalyn Walsh
McLean (1886–1948) exemplified this trend. Friend of first lady
Florence Harding and owner of the Hope diamond, McLean
lived a rags-to-riches story, the riches materializing when she
married newspaper heir Ted B. McLean. About reports of fast
driving on their honeymoon she said, "Dosed with laudanum
and whiskey, I did not care about the risk so long as we were not
riding in the other fellow's dust." In 1905, she was put on morphine to counter pains resulting from a car accident and
remained on morphine for much of the rest of her life.[31]

I have often seen fashionable people with a regular arsenal of little injecting instruments, who, thanks to their medical men, had always at their disposal a solution of morphia strong enough to poison them. Ladies even, belonging to the most elegant classes of society, go so far as to show their good taste in the jewels which they order to conceal a little syringe and artistically made bottles, which are destined to hold the solution which enchants them!—Dr. Zambaco (c. 1887)

By the last decade of the 1800s, attitudes towards opium use were changing. Drug addiction, now recognized, was debated and denounced; opium smoking was being legislated out of visible existence, especially in North America; patent medicines and their creators were under fire—1906 saw the passing of laws in Britain and the United States regulating such medicines. Yet in 1908, the San Francisco *Examiner* ran a full-page exposé of bejewelled morphine kits—complete with syringes and vials—available in fashionable stores in New York. Titled "Has It Come to This?" the article quivered with outrage: "The inference is that rich and fashionable women now receive at the most sacred Christmas season congratulatory gifts, which mark their enslavement to one of the most degrading and ruinous of vices." The cases cost from $135 to $500, but the high prices were no deterrent; one especially hollow-eyed woman was even seen to order two.[33]

That such a trend would trickle down to the poor is no surprise. Upton Sinclair wrote of morphine addiction in early 1900s Chicago. In his novel *The Jungle* (1906), Marija, a poor immigrant woman driven to prostitution declares, "The madame always gives them dope when they first come, and they learn to like it; or else they take it for headaches and such things,

Morphine kits, c. 1901–20. Designed for discretion, kits holding a syringe, needles and vials were disguised as lighters, cigarette cases and flasks. The kit at bottom right was featured in the 1908 San Francisco *Examiner* article "Has It Come to This?" *Far right:* a device for holding vials and a syringe secure. Top left and bottom right, courtesy Colin Schebek

Antic Hay A passerby notices Mrs. Viveash, who is mumbling to herself on the street:
"Poor thing, he thought, poor young thing. Talking to herself. Must be cracked, must be off her head. Or perhaps she took drugs. That was more likely: that was much more likely. Most of them did nowadays. Vicious young women. Lesbians, drug-fiends, nymphomaniacs, dipsos—thoroughly vicious, nowadays, thoroughly vicious. He arrived at his club in an excellent temper."[32]

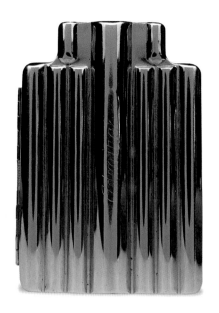

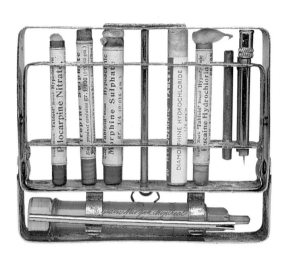

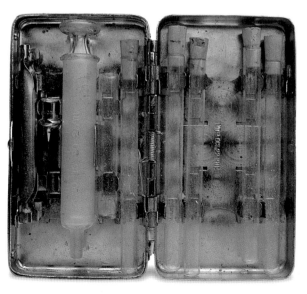

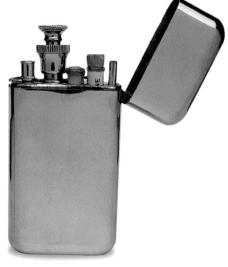

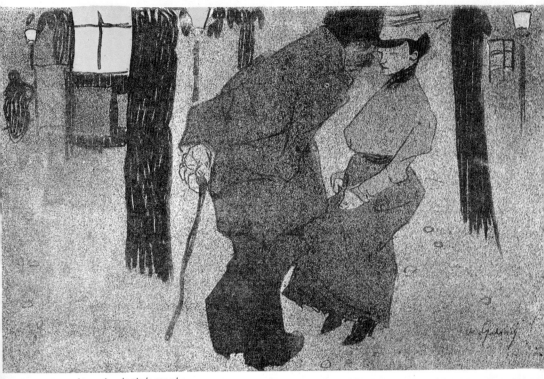

— ... *Je suis dactylographe...*
— *Menteuse !... Faites voir vos piqûres d'aiguille.*

and get the habit that way. I've got it, I know; I've tried to quit, but I never will while I'm here."[34]

Lower- and middle-class men were by no means exempt from this form of addiction, but their addictions were spread over a far wider field. Men had recourse to drinking along with cigarette and even opium smoking, behaviour that most women were not permitted to indulge in, unless covertly. Medical use of morphine, along with other opium medicines, was for them, at least for a while, a legitimate means of escape.

La Police: II. A plain-clothed policeman confronts a woman whom he suspects to be a prostitute and drug addict. The caption reads: " 'I'm a typist.' 'Liar! Show me your needle marks.' " Drawing by Galanis, from *L'Assiette au beurre,* 30 May 1903, 1914.

**The diary of an opium
cure** "At the clinic, at five
o'clock, the old bull-dog who
is dying is given a fatal injection of morphine. One hour
later he is playing in the
garden, jumping and rolling
about. The following day, at
five, he scratched at the
doctor's door and asked for
his injection."—Jean
Cocteau[35]

Léon Daudet. Drawing by Don,
reprinted in Eugène Montfort, *Vingt-
cinq ans de littérature française*, Paris:
Librairie de France, vol. I, 1920, 265.

La Lutte "I was . . . trying
to think of nothing, not easy
when the word opium is
engraved in every one of our
cells in letters of fire."[36]

Morphine addiction in the medical profession was significant enough to draw attention; though the problem was global,
it seemed especially severe in France, no doubt because of the
writings of Léon Daudet and Oscar Jennings, the latter a one-
time morphine-addicted doctor. Doctors had a steady supply of
drugs, their hours were long, the conditions were stressful and
they saw the relief that morphine could provide firsthand.
Jennings reported in his book *The Morphia Habit* (1909) a claim
that "20 per cent. of the mortality amongst medical men was due
to morphino-mania."[37]

Léon Daudet was a doctor, journalist, novelist and reactionary and
never took opium, preferring
instead the refinements of two and a
half bottles of wine a day.[38] He
denounced drugs in his novel *La
Lutte (The Struggle)* (1907), which
was based on his experiences as an
intern. The hero is a young doctor
with a bright future who suddenly
discovers that he's tubercular.
Desperate for relief, he takes mor-

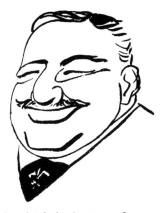

phine. The novel's upbeat ending—it's subtitled *The Story of a
Cure*—contrasts with Russian author Mikhail Bulgakov's tragic
short story "Morphine," about morphine-addicted physician
Polyakov, who takes the drug, first for stomach trouble, then for
anguish over a failed love affair.

Hungarian doctor/writer Géza Csáth began using opium in
1909 and a year later was injecting morphine. After serving in
World War I he became unhinged, started carrying knives, had

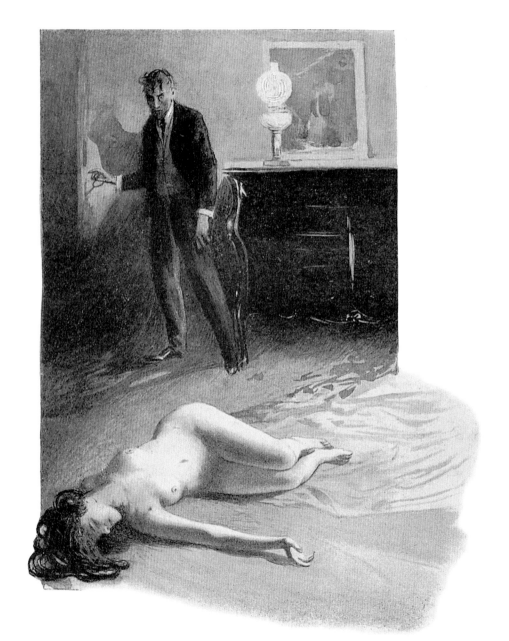

La Morphine, Victorien du Saussay. Raoul, the morphinomane, has attacked his wife, Blanche, because she has hidden money from him. Illustration by Manuel Orazi. Paris: Albert Méricant, n.d.

Morphine, 1891

Captain Pontaillac has just openly injected morphine into his leg at the Café de la Paix, in front of shocked friends. Luce Molday grabs his syringe—often called a Pravaz in France—and passes it to Major Lapouge:

" 'I won't give this back to you, Captain! I'll crush it under my heel!' exclaimed Lapouge, standing.

" 'Don't bother yourself about it, Major; I've had my shot. There's another Pravaz in my pocket, and I have fourteen at home.' "[39]

his family followed by detectives and then shot his wife in front of their daughter. He was placed in an insane asylum from which he escaped. When caught, he swallowed poison and died. His short story "Opium" is an apologia for his weakness, and in diary passages from 1913, he bemoans his addiction: "To commit sin, to harm myself without enjoying it, this is the bitter thought tormenting me. If I had a gun near me, at times like this, I would blow my brains out, right away."[40]

Like laudanum, morphine was written of as part of the lives of people from all walks of life, especially by French novelists and especially in the decadent 1890s. Alphonse Daudet worked his knowledge of morphine into a brief passage in his damning novel of religious fervour, L'Évangeliste (1883). Novelist and playwright Rachilde acknowledged morphine addiction in her play Madame La Mort (1891). Les Imprudences de Peggy (n.d.), by Meg Villar and Colette's ex-husband Willy, was a satire of Colette and her circle, featuring a morphine-addicted baroness, a direct stab at Colette's lover Missy.[41]

Then there were the novels that damned both morphine and decadence. Noris (1883) by Jules Claretie, Morphine (1891) by Jean-Louis Dubut de Laforest, La Possédés de la morphine (1892) by Maurice Talmeyr, La Comtesse Morphine (1885) by Marcel Mallat de Bassilan and La Morphine (n.d.) by Victorien du Saussay were fervently anti-morphine.

In La Morphine, a stark novel of addiction, failed cures, incest, indecent exposure and adultery, desperate morphine addict Raoul lives in abject poverty with his wife, Blanche. When Blanche manages to hold on to a few sous for house-keeping expenses, Raoul beats her senseless to get it. His sister Thérèse, a classy call girl, is a morphine dabbler, but his other two sisters, low-class prostitutes Antoinette and Jacqueline, are what were known as *adeptes*, addicted. In one charming scene of family intimacy, Raoul, Antoinette and Jacqueline share Raoul's syringe, a Christmas present from the thoughtful Thérèse. Du Saussay ends the book with a plea to the youth of France to bring their noble country back to its former drug-free glory.

Morphine is the instrument of murder in the Fantômas novel called *Le Cercueil vide (The Empty Coffin)*. The story begins in surgeon Paul Drop's near-bankrupt clinic with the death of one of his rich female patients. Her nephew, Pedro Corales, is ecstatic and grateful, as he is heir to her vast fortune, which he proceeds to blow on a destructive drug habit. When he begs Drop for morphine, an associate of the doctor's, the businessman Minias, convinces Drop to supply it. Minias administers the morphine himself, ensuring that Corales, who just happens to have a wad of francs stuffed into his pocket, dies from an overdose. Minias, who turns out to be Fantômas, that evil genius of disguise, naturally helps himself to the money.

Morphine murders weren't limited to fiction. French doctor Edme-Samuel Castaing went on trial in 1823, accused of poisoning his friend Claude-Auguste Ballet to inherit the Ballet family's fortune. When the death was investigated, it was discovered that Ballet's father, mother, uncle and brother had also died under suspicious circumstances, that Castaing had purchased considerable amounts of morphine shortly before Ballet died and that he'd made a similar purchase in advance of Ballet's brother Hippolyte's death. In spite of his protestations of innocence, Castaing was condemned to lose his head; Alexandre Dumas wrote the execution into his novel *The Count of Monte Cristo* (1844–46). In 1907, Laurent Tailhade revived the story and

La Morphine "My eyes are troubled, my senses awaken, irresistible torments are kindled in me . . . Oh! I can't bear it, I'm crazy, but, so what! . . . it's my turn, the morphine! . . . Oh! Morphine, the divine poison which makes us equal with the gods!"—Thérèse, *La Morphine*[42]

Little Lady of the Big House, 1916 Jack London, who began taking morphine around 1908, wrote a morphine mercy killing into his novel *The Little Lady of the Big House*. In this story, Paula has shot herself and is revived briefly by a doctor before being given a lethal injection of morphine:
" 'Sleepy, sleepy,' [Paula] twittered in mimicry of drowsy birds. 'I am ready, doctor. Stretch the skin tight first. You know I don't like to be hurt.' "[43]

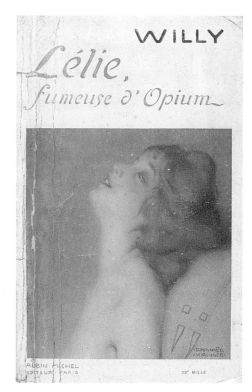

Lélie, fumeuse d'opium by Willy (pseudonym of Henry Gauthier-Villars) and Paul-Jean Toulet. Willy did not likely use drugs, but Toulet was an inveterate opium smoker. Cover by Raphaël Kirchner. Paris: Albin Michel, 1911.

added details of the actual poisoning. His account and Dumas's differ though, in that Tailhade suggests that the murder for which Castaing was arrested was Hippolyte's, not Claude-Auguste's.[44]

Thomas Griffiths Wainewright, English dandy, rake, forger, artist and critic, was found guilty of poisoning a string of relatives, commencing with his uncle in 1828, possibly with a strychnine and morphine mix. He was shipped off to Tasmania for his crimes. Oscar Wilde wrote that when Wainewright was refused a pardon "the associate of Coleridge consoled himself by making those marvelous *Paradis Artificiels* whose secret is only known to the eaters of opium."[45]

A later case of poisoning involved Colette's first husband, Willy, who was suspected, though never charged, of poisoning—out of mercy— his son's sick mother, Germaine Servat, in 1892. The suspicion arose after Willy asked Colette's brother Achille, who was a doctor, how much morphine would be fatal; Achille subsequently noticed that a vial of morphine was missing.[46]

By the turn of the century, people who consumed morphine in its recognizable forms knew they were taking risks. As we'll see in the next chapter, however, there were a hundreds of ways to take opium without realizing it.

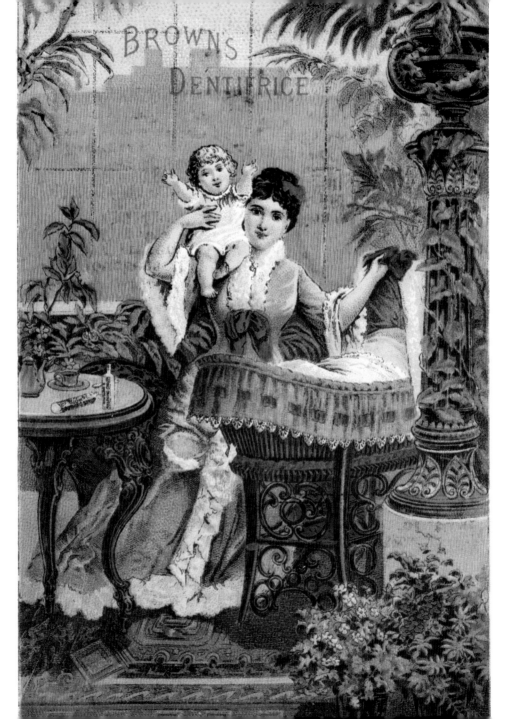

I Like It! I Want It!

PATENT MEDICINES
FROM CRADLE TO GRAVE

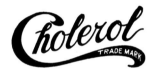

This page, top: Piso's, which came in green bottles, contained *Cannabis indica* and morphine sulfate up to at least 1902, even though the manufacturer declared it morphine and opium free by 1872.[1] *Bottom:* Cholerol, containing opium, was specifically prescribed for diarrhoea.

Facing page: Although this trade card is for Brown's Dentifrice, it was originally distributed for Mrs. Winslow's Soothing Syrup and shows a labelled bottle of the syrup on the table.

"It Never Fails!" "Relieves Little Sufferers at Once," "Perfectly Harmless," "Saved My Life."

These fabulous claims were made by American patent medicine companies in the 1880s and '90s, when medical hucksterism hit a peak. They offered cures for everything from asthma to yellow fever and exploited sufferers shamelessly, lacing their medicines with habit-forming substances such as opium and alcohol. I have identified almost three hundred patent medicines containing opium; there were probably many more.

Patent medicines, which were almost never patented, appealed to those at the bottom of the social heap. They were easily available and relatively cheap and often seemed effective if they contained a powerful substance like opium. They could also be self-administered, an advantage, perhaps, in an age when doctors were not only expensive but at times downright dangerous.

Known more accurately as proprietary medicines, patent medicines were shrouded in secrecy. Their creators avoided the patent process that required them to reveal the sometimes fraudulent, sometime hazardous, and always questionable contents of their "miracle" cures and instead chose to protect their trademark. The phrase "patent medicine" became a misnomer and a catchall. This doesn't mean there were no truly patented medicines: the first such patent in Britain was taken out in either 1698 or 1711 and in the United States in the 1790s. One of the first patents for opium medicine was granted in 1726 to the maker of Dr. Bateman's Pectoral Drops, a tincture of gambir and opium.[2]

What was the dividing line between legitimate and quack medicines? The distinctions were vague, especially since some medicines now considered fraudulent were sold by pharmacists. Two such opium medicines included in the *London Pharmacopœia* were Daffy's Elixir, consisting of opium and senna, and Matthew's Pills, made of opium and soap.[3] Opium, and after 1820, morphine, was mixed with everything imaginable: mercury, hashish, cayenne pepper, ether, chloroform, belladonna, whisky, wine and brandy.

Of the early opium nostrums, Godfrey's Cordial and Dover's Powder are among the most interesting. Godfrey's, made of sassafras, molasses and laudanum, was a popular household remedy by 1722. According to its makers, it could cure just about anything: colic, fever, measles, restlessness and smallpox, though teething became its main focus. To give an idea of the amounts dispensed, in 1808 a Nottingham chemist sold 200 pounds of opium and 600 pints of Godfrey's; another, in Long Sutton, Lincolnshire (population 6,000), sold 25½ gallons (204 pints) of Godfrey's in 1871.[4]

The original formula for Dover's was published in Thomas Dover's *The Ancient Physician's Legacy to his Country* (1742). A one-time apprentice of Thomas Sydenham, Dover had been a South Seas adventurer before turning to medicine. He was known as "The Quicksilver Doctor" because he freely prescribed mercury.[5] In his book, Dover's Powder is specified as a cure for gout—though it was soon used for many ailments, including teething. Dover declared that he "very much" disliked opium and admitted that

Chlorodyne One of the most pernicious yet useful drugs ever devised, chlorodyne contained chloroform, morphine and alcohol. Developed to combat the effects of cholera and dysentery, it was also used against neuralgia, gout, cancer, toothache, colds, fever and rheumatism. By 1885 there were many variations; Dr. Chase's (1898) recipe included "stronger ether, stronger alcohol and muriate of morphia." Beasley's listed Dr. Ogden's recipe, which also had "resin of Indian hemp." Menthol, peppermint, licorice and molasses gave it flavour.

Facing page, left: Dr. J. Collis Browne's Chlorodyne ads appeared in almanacs and newspapers. *The Graphic,* 1888.

Facing page, right: Freeman's Chlorodyne logo. Freeman's was sued by Dr. J. Collis Browne's, and apparently won the suit, according to their ads in *Whitacker's Almanack,* 1879.

some Apothecaries have desired their Patients to make their Wills, and settle their Affairs, before they venture upon so large a Dose as I have recommended, which is from Forty to Seventy Grains. As monstrous as they may represent this, I can produce undeniable Proofs, where a Patient of mine has taken no less a Quantity than an Hundred Grains, and yet has appear'd abroad the next Day.[6]

A later arrival to the medicine scene was Dr. J. Collis Browne's Chlorodyne, a mix of chloroform, morphine and "other ingredients." Created in 1856 by Dr. Browne, "late of the Army Medical Staff," for those serving in India, chlorodyne was a powerful antidote to diarrhoea, indispensable for sufferers of cholera and dysentery and thus popular with travellers. In Maud Diver's novel *The Great Amulet* (1913) about life in colonial India, chlorodyne is described as sweet, with a "strong sickly odour."[7]

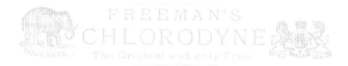

J. Collis Browne was up against several other chlorodyne makers, as recipes for this and other popular elixirs did not remain secret for long. Competitors, whether it was the fellow next door trying out a new angle or a pharmacist seeking higher profits, tested the remedies, then sold the recipes in formularies or "receipt" books. A pharmacist armed with one of these handy books could mix his own tonics, selling them in bottles specially stamped with his store's name or in refilled bottles of recognized brands.

(US 1897); Stoke's Expectorant (US c. 1926); Stowell's Cold Remedy

There were also receipt books for the family bookshelf. *Richardson's Medicology* (1903), *Dr. Chase's Recipes, or Information for Everybody* (many editions) and *Dr. Mintie's* (1878) gave democratic access to many drugs. Their recipes, aimed at the layperson, are intimidating today; amounts were listed in incomprehensible measures such as drams, scruples and minims or in mind-boggling quantities; for instance, Dr. Chase's Analgesic called for 20 pounds of powdered guaiac, 2 pounds of gum camphor, 6 pounds of powdered cayenne pepper, 1 to 3 pounds of powdered opium and 32 gallons of alcohol. Many of the ingredients were exotic: myrhh, tolu, squibbs; or deadly: belladonna, mercury, lead, opium. Dosages were often vague; Compound Syrup of White Pine, for example, was made with 3 to 16 grains of morphia, and the suggested dose was 3 to 4 teaspoons per day.[9]

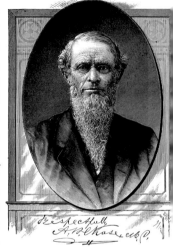

Some medicines seemed designed to eliminate the patient rather than the affliction. Richardson's bed-wetting cure contained strychnine, cantharides (Spanish fly) and morphine. Just three pills a day was guaranteed to stop incontinence. Others had the narcotic angle thoroughly covered. Hamlin's Cough Syrup was made up of ipecac, antimony, Syrup of Wild Cherry, and 12 grains of acetate of morphia, but Syrup of Wild Cherry itself contained 8 grains of sulfate of morphia.[10] Piso's Consumption Cure, seeking effectiveness in variety, was made up of *Cannabis indica*, morphine and alcohol.

Above: Dr. A.W. Chase. This portrait appeared in *Dr. Chase's Receipt Book and Household Physician, or Practical Knowledge for the People*, published after his death in 1898. Chase claimed medical training at the Cincinnati Eclectic College of Medicine then at the University of Michigan. In his own words, he was "placed . . . at the head of his profession in the State of Michigan and his fame as a wonderfully successful physician spread abroad."[8]

Left: Piso's Cure for Consumption, packaging detail, n.d.

Opium eased the pains of teething and controlled diarrhoea brought on by weaning, and it was a cheap babysitter for poor women who worked outside the home. Mothers could dose their babies and leave them, knowing they would sleep through the day. Furthermore, a child fed opium loses its appetite, another benefit for poor families who couldn't afford to feed their offspring properly. Dosed children became jaundiced and thin, their heads seemingly overlarge for their weak bodies.

Testifying that childhood soothing syrups were partly responsible for his opium addiction, William Cobbe wrote that he had been given paregoric, Godfrey's, Dr. Bateman's and laudanum "whenever lamentations from any cause evoked the spectre of impossible disease." He claimed that this habit "gave to the physical cells an appetite which they never lost."[11]

Novelists worked opium syrups into their stories. In Charlotte Yonge's novel *The Three Brides* (1850), wealthy mother Lady Rosamond becomes hysterical after a day at the races when she discovers her baby's nurse soothing the child with an opiate. Her nonchalant doctor tells her that "it only remains to be proved whether an aristocratic baby can bear popular treatment. I dare say some hundred unlucky infants have been lugged out to the racecourse to-day, and come back squalling their hearts out with

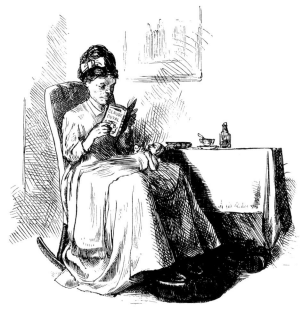

As his nurse reads the latest pot-boiler by Claude Duval, her charge lies in her lap, stupefied by a soothing syrup. Uncredited sketch from "The Seven Ages of Man," in *Harper's Weekly*, 11 October 1873, 912.

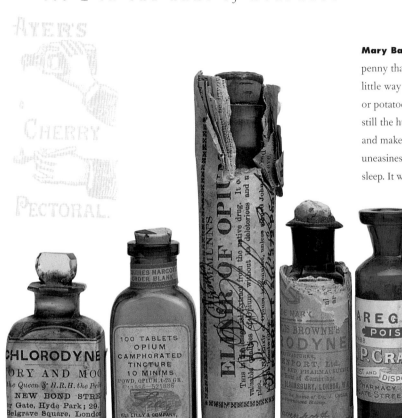

Mary Barton "Many a penny that would have gone little way enough in oatmeal or potatoes, bought opium to still the hungry little ones, and make them forget their uneasiness in heavy troubled sleep. It was mother's mercy."[12]

Above: A selection of opium medicines used against coughs, colds, diarrhoea, teething and innumerable other maladies. *From left to right:* Savory and Moore Chlorodyne, Eli Lilly Camphorated Tincture of Opium Tablets, McMunn's Elixir of Opium, Dr. J. Collis Browne's Chlorodyne, Paregoric, Pulverized Opium Tablets. *Top left and bottom right:* From an almanac advertising Ayer's Cherry Pectoral and Ayer's Pills.

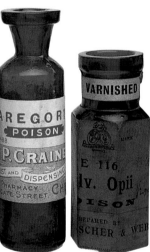

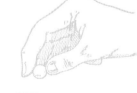

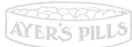

Taylor's Sweet Gum and Mullein Compound (US 1909); Teasdale's Chlorodyne (GB 1859); Theriaca Andromachi aka

Amelia (Emmy) catches her mother feeding Daffy's Elixir to her baby, Georgy, in W. M. Thackeray's *Vanity Fair.* Illustration by the author, vol. II, 247.

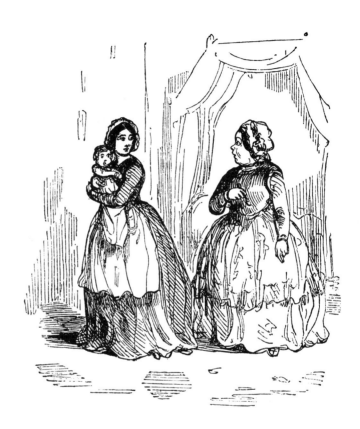

Daffy's

"'I will not have baby poisoned, mamma,' cried Emmy, rocking the infant about violently with both her arms round him, and turning with flashing eyes at her mother . . . 'He shall not have any medicine but that which Mr. Pestler sends for him. He told me that Daffy's Elixir was poison.'"—*Vanity Fair*[13]

Baby killer

One calculation determined that on the basis of 750,000 bottles of Mrs. Winslow's sold annually in the United States, each with an average of ¾ grain of morphine, a total of 562,500 grains . . . was "enough to kill a half million infants not accustomed to its use."[14]

fatigue and hunger, and I'll be bound that nine-tenths are lulled with this very sedative, and will be none the worse." In *Vanity Fair*, Mrs. Sedly gives a shot of Daffy's to her grandson Georgy, and in *Mary Barton*, Manchester mothers dose their babies.[15]

Of the soothing syrups, none reached the success attained by the American product Mrs. Winslow's. Sold from 1830 until at least 1910, this potent teething elixir was made from sugar syrup,

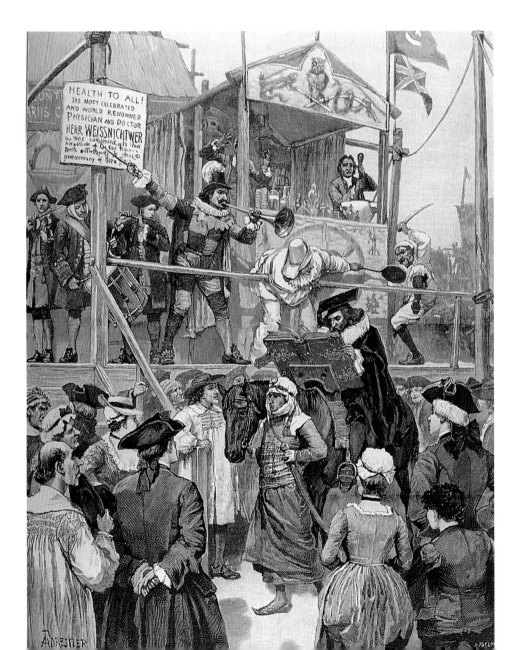

HEALTH TO ALL!
THE MOST CELEBRATED
AND WORLD RENOWNED
PHYSICIAN AND DOCTOR
HERR WEISSNICHTWER

Facing page: "Room for the Doctor, Gentlemen." A nineteenth-century rendition of a medieval fair. Drawing by A. Forestier, engraving by R. Taylor. *Illustrated London News,* 4 September 1886, 245.

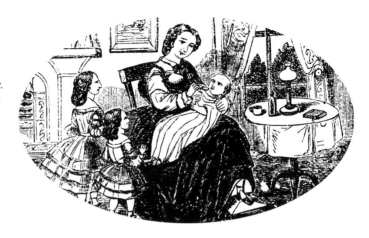

This page: Mrs. Winslow's Domestic Receipt Book. Used to promote Mrs. Winslow's, Brown's Bronchial Troches, Brown's Vermifuge Comfits, Brown's Household Panacea and Brown's Dentifrice, 1877.

Paregoric in the nursery

"*Paregoric,* that household bane so empirically and yet so lavishly dispensed by imprudent mothers, whether for its supposed prophylactic virtue, has been, as an instrument of retributive evil, the very Nemesis of the nursery."—Calkins[16]

fennel, anise, caraway, alcohol and morphine sulfate. *Nostrums* (1911) attributed a number of deaths to the potion for the years 1906–10.[17]

Up to the early 1900s many of the most popular teething remedies, in addition to Godfrey's and Mrs. Winslow's, contained morphine or opium. And some also contained scandalous amounts of alcohol. Battley's Sedative Solution called for opium and three types of alcohol. Ingham's Vegetable Expectorant Nervine Pain Extractor, containing opium and 86 per cent alcohol, claimed, "If sick it will do good; if well it will do no harm."[18]

Medical quacks had begun peddling their nostrums at the large medieval fairs throughout Europe, a tradition that persevered into the twentieth century and also spread to North America. Advertising started with the printed handbill but really took off with the appearance of newspapers. In the late 1700s, a London paper such as the *Daily Post* would devote almost a full page in an edition of four pages to medicinal advertisements.

The publicized medicaments were sold at apothecary shops as well as at toy shops, booksellers, coffeehouses and by "the Gentlewoman at the two Blue Posts in Haydon-Yard." By the mid-1700s, American nostrums were also available at such unapothecary-sounding places as those of hairdressers, post-masters and tailors.[20]

As time passed, medicine ads claimed that a scientific break-through had been made or that the secret key ingredient had been discovered in a remote part of the world, the Sandwich Islands, for instance.[21] Many nostrum makers called themselves Doctor; others appealed to the wisdom of age with monikers such as Grandmother. Still others—Professor C. E. Matthai's Victory and Thomas's Electric Oil come to mind—adopted a scientific approach.

Some makers promised narcotic-free concoctions because, even though consumption of opiates was commonplace, there were still warnings, especially in newspapers and novels, about their effects. So, if a medicine was potent but benign, patients could rest easy, happily duped that their well-being was brought about by a dose of a "purely vegetable compound" and not by alcohol, morphine or cocaine. Hodnett's Gem Soothing Syrup (4 4/5 grains opium/ounce, 4 per cent alcohol) and Dr. Fahrney's Teething Syrup (0.126 grains morphine/ounce, 8 per cent alcohol) both made such false claims.[22]

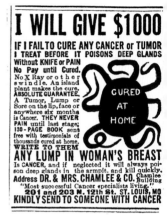

Dr. Chamlee Cancer Cure, Prep. #2. One of the most heinous crimes committed by nineteenth-century quacks was the claim that their worthless tonics could cure cancer. This advertisement for a "cure" containing opium as well as 22 per cent alcohol was reprinted in *Nostrums and Quackery*, 1911, 33.

KEATING'S COUGH LOZENGES are daily recommended by the Faculty for their certain cure of Coughs, Asthma, Bronchitis. One Lozenge alone gives relief, they contain no opium nor any deleterious drug. Sold by all Chemists, in Boxes, 1s. 1½d., and Tins, 2s. 9d. each.

Keating's Cough Lozenges, produced at least as early as 1876, claimed "no opium," but analysts for *Nostrums and Quackery*, 1911, and *Secret Remedies* found morphine.[19]

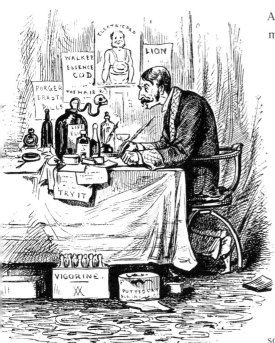

Cartoon lampooning "Lord Gryle," who makes a living by writing testimonials for quack medicine ads. Grenville-Murray, *Side-Lights of English Society*. London: Vizetelly, 1883, 278.

Advertising became more innovative. Patent medicine companies distributed collectible trade cards beginning in the 1820s and peaking in the 1880s. Early examples showed peaceful rural or historical scenes; the later ones pulled off the gloves: Mrs. Winslow's issued a series of chromolithographs featuring loving mothers soaking their babies in alcohol and morphine sulfate. They also produced almanacs and instructional booklets filled with helpful hints and the diseases to be vanquished by the featured brand. Dr. Pierce's printed a pamphlet on pelvic diseases for women only; Mrs. Winslow's interspersed recipes for hotcakes and puddings with shaming denunciations of mothers who didn't have its soothing syrup on hand; Dr. Chase shared formulas for the elixirs of other quacks. And that was just the start; brand names were painted in letters several feet high onto the sides of barns; men sporting sandwich boards walked city streets; promotional merchandise such as Monell's Teething Syrup clocks was distributed to druggists; and itinerant quacks, regularly hopping from town to town, skillfully roped in suckers.[23]

French opium advertising was more restrained, but for coca tonic aperitifs such as Vin Mariani and absinthe, France surpassed the excesses of Britain and America. Vin Mariani was promoted in booklets and ads and, most memorably, through

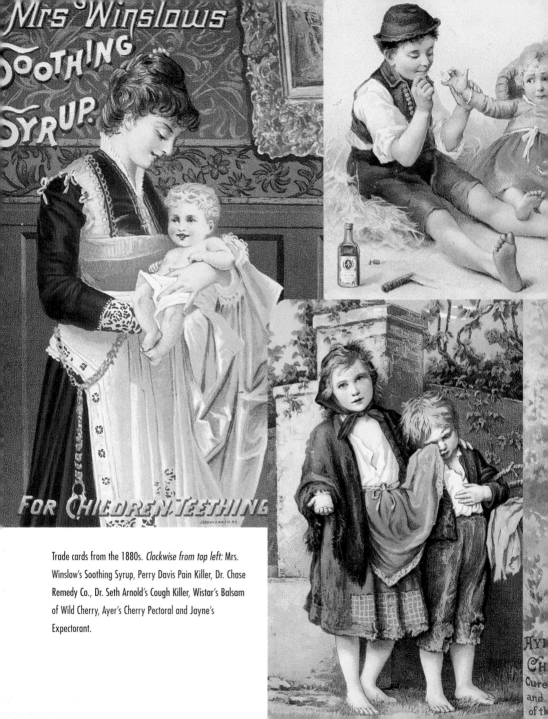

Trade cards from the 1880s. *Clockwise from top left:* Mrs. Winslow's Soothing Syrup, Perry Davis Pain Killer, Dr. Chase Remedy Co., Dr. Seth Arnold's Cough Killer, Wistar's Balsam of Wild Cherry, Ayer's Cherry Pectoral and Jayne's Expectorant.

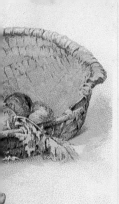

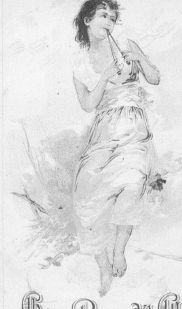

Gate Remedy Co.
C·H·I·C·A·G·O

"Don't cry
smart a moment; the
KILLER will soon take
the soreness away."

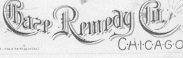

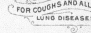

WISTAR'S BALSAM OF
WILD CHERRY
FOR COUGHS AND ALL
LUNG DISEASES

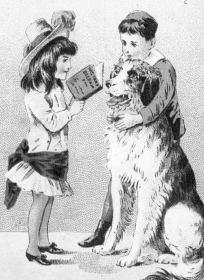

ECTORAL

ughs,

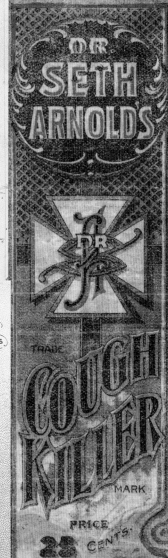

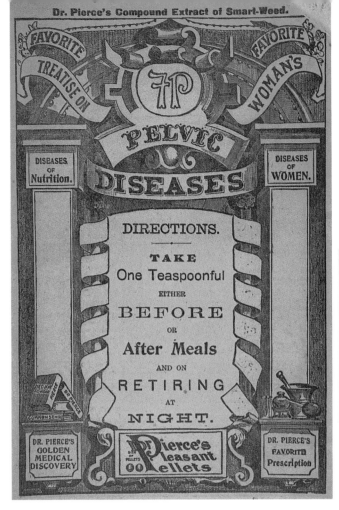

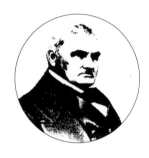

Top: Portrait of Perry Davis, from packaging for Perry Davis Pain Killer. On the market from 1830 until about 1956, during the late 1800s it was made from myrhh, capsicum, opium, benzoin, guaiac and alcohol.[24]

Above: Mrs. Winslow's advertising in English, German and French.

Left: Dr. Pierce's Almanac, c. 1890.

posters featuring deliriously happy women. Absinthe, an alcoholic drink containing wormwood, was not only widely advertised but also immortalized by Picasso, Toulouse-Lautrec and Degas. This preference didn't stop American nostrum purveyors from invading the continent; Mrs. Winslow's, Ayer's and Perry Davis advertised widely in French and German and found success worldwide.

On your own "God seems to help a man in getting out of every difficulty but opium. There you have to *claw* your way out over red-hot coals on your hands and knees, and drag yourself by main strength through the burning dungeon-bars."—Anonymous addict[25]

Hammett and the cure

In *The Dain Curse*, Hammett's nameless op tries to cure Gabrielle Dain of her morphine habit:

"'I want,' I told Vic, 'fifty grains of M. and eight of those calomel-ipecac-atropine-strychnine-cascara shots. I'll have somebody from the agency pick up the package to-night . . .'

"'If you say so, but if you kill anybody with it don't tell them where you got the stuff.'"[26]

No matter how free they claimed to be, opium never relinquished its hold on either De Quincey or Coleridge, or on a host of other addicts. These failures, however, didn't stop physicians, social do-gooders and quack medicine men from trying to promote their own brands of opium cures.

By the beginning of the twentieth century, there was a growing sense that opium had permeated the West and governments began instituting controls on all narcotics. This move opened up new entrepreneurial opportunities: sanitariums offered the latest in sure-fire withdrawal techniques that rarely worked; opium cures, deceptively laced with opium or morphine, were sold through newspaper advertising.

De Quincey had already shared with his readers the torture of trying to free himself from dependence. He rejoiced that in 1816 he suddenly dropped his consumption from a high of eight thousand drops a day to *only* one thousand and enthused that "the process of weaning one's self from the deep bondage of opium, by many people viewed with despairing eyes, is . . . a possible achievement, and one which grows easier in every stage of its progress."[27]

But by the end of the century, no one much believed in De Quincey's kind of cure and elixirs flourished, provoking journalist Samuel Hopkins Adams (*Collier's*, 1906) and the editors of *Nostrums and Quackery* (1911) to write exposés of the morphine-cure industry. Any amount of morphine in a morphine cure would be alarming, but many of the treatments they fingered contained as much as 2 grains of morphine per dose. O. P. Coats dished out 2½ grains; Habitina, not taking any chances, contained 8 grains of morphine sulfate and 4 grains of heroin hydrochloride. The Coblentz Cure provided 20 grains of morphine a day—more than many addicts would have been accustomed to taking.* The names were as reassuring as the elixirs that had helped create the addictions: Carney Common Sense Opiate Cure, Dr. J. C. Hoffman Cure, Drug Crave Crusade, Morphina-Cura, St. Anne's Morphin Cure and Hopeine, which had nothing to do with hope; it was morphine "perfumed and slightly coloured by hops."[29]

Little ads offering complete mail-order cures in ten to thirty days for as little as $2.00 were scattered throughout weeklies such as *Harper's* and *Frank Leslie's*. The Humane Remedy gave out free trial samples, as did the St. James Society, along with a statement that their medicine contained the GREAT VITAL PRINCIPAL. Sears retailed the Reliable Cure from the Opium and Morphia Habit—active ingredient undisclosed.

Other chemical battles against opium addiction included atropine, the nonaddicting alkaloid from *Atropa belladonna; Cannabis indica*, codeine, chloral and heroin. Morphine addict Ernest von Fleischl-Marxow had cause to regret his friendship with Sigmund Freud when the psychiatrist recommended cocaine as a cure and von Fleischl-Marxow became hopelessly addicted to cocaine.[30]

Oscar Jennings wrote of his attempts to shake off morphine addiction, bemoaning "quack remedies containing nothing but morphia, which may become endowed with a potency which is the measure at the time of the credulity of the dupe who takes them and of the cleverness of those who apply in this manner psychology to trade." Jennings tried a number of medicines, including dionine, hyoscine and atropine, but preferred the idea

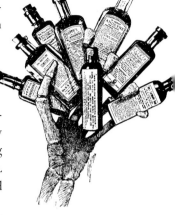

Above: "Baby Killer" from *Nostrums and Quackery,* 1911, 317.

Facing page: Dope: Adventures of David Dare by Earle Albert Rowell. David Dare thwarts conniving narcotic smugglers. The girl on the cover of this self-righteous semi-fictional novel is undergoing withdrawal. The caption inside the book reads "A victim of the wolves of society. This . . . shows the effort of a new addict to break the spell of the drug upon her."[28] Uncredited cover art, 1937.

* According to Adams, a normal dose of morphine in grains was 0.175; a relatively strong dose would be 0.25 grains of morphine.[31]

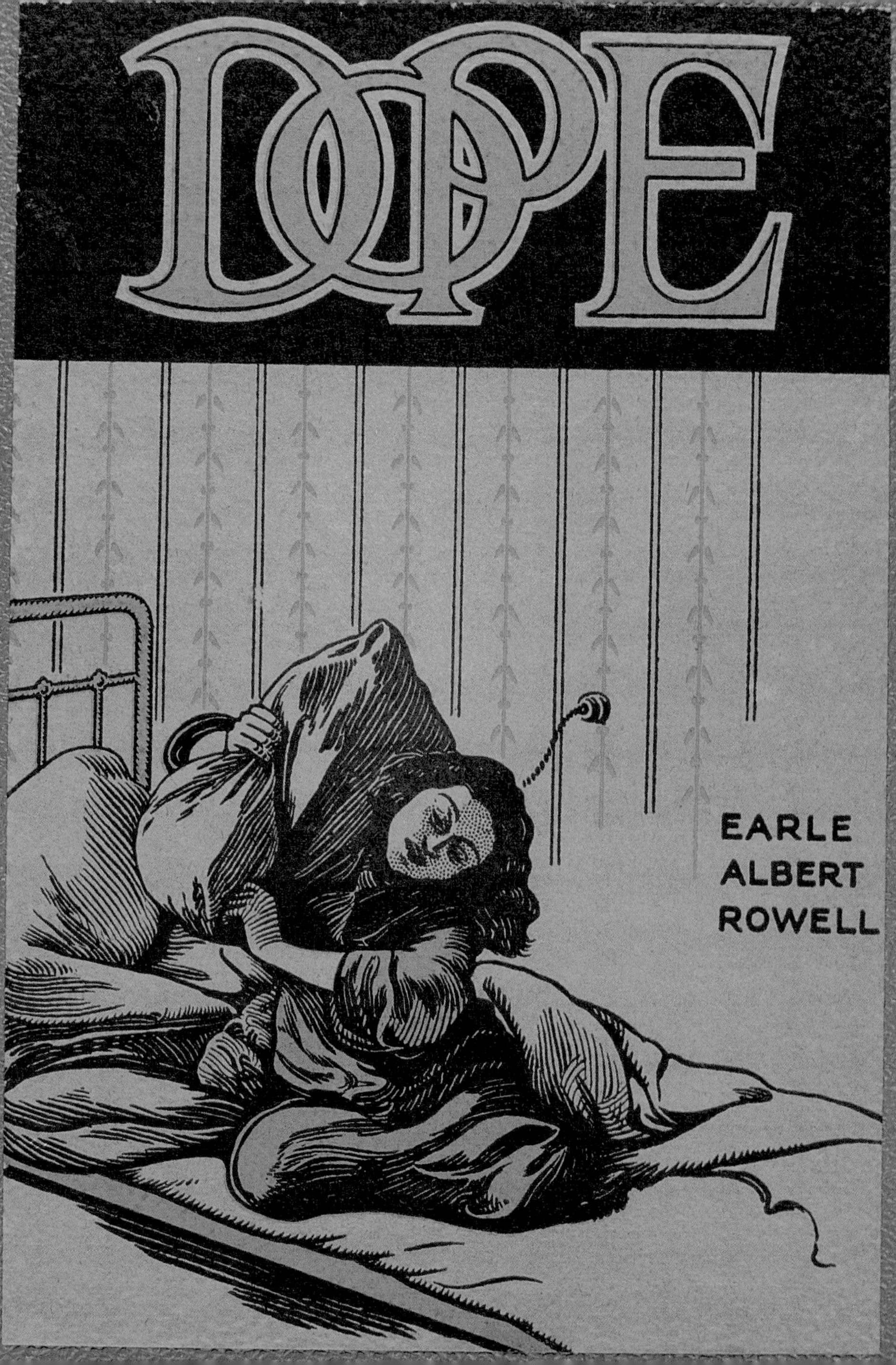
DOPE
EARLE
ALBERT
ROWELL

Coblentz cure "Do not take every cure you see advertised, for how easy it is to disguise the drug under the garb of a new cure and beguile the poor, unsuspecting victim into the belief of being cured while all the time he is taking the drug under a different name."—Promotional claim (According to *Nostrums and Quackery*, 1911, a twenty-four-hour course of the Coblentz cure would furnish 20 grains of morphine.)

of establishing favourable conditions such as "the love of a good woman."[32]

Horace Day espoused a De Quincey–style cure, at that time called slow-reduction. Jennings quoted Dr. M. Sollier, who likened it to cutting off a dog's tail by inches. Jennings didn't think much of the other extreme either, quoting Dr. Grover Burnett, who dismissed rapid withdrawal as "a method that extinguishes the patient's mental lights and thrusts him into a tophetic crucible that would make hell a paradise and the accepted purgatory without candles an oasis in Sahara!"[33]

Thanks to the crackdown on patent medicine manufacturers, the general populace was weaned off opium medicines; many people continued to take their medicines, now opium free, and when they realized that the medicines were no longer as effective, they stopped taking them. Patent medicines were less relevant anyway; standards of living were steadily improving; other, nonaddictive pain-killing medicines were becoming available; and there had been a backlash when reports such as Adams's series in *Collier's* revealed the extent to which the West was poisoning itself. This is not to say that patent medicines disappeared; they just became less potent and more accountable. Desperate people still sought cures for incurable ailments: above all, faith healers established their popularity.

In the '30s you could write away for the Keeley Cure for Tobacco, Natural Eyesight devices, drugless ulcer treatments and prostate massagers; in the '50s, for antidiabetic foot cream, varicose vein eradicators and weight-loss candies; and in the '90s, any number of hair-renew lotions, diet foods and impotence vanquishers. Although opium is no longer part of it, the story of patent medicines clearly has not yet come to a close.

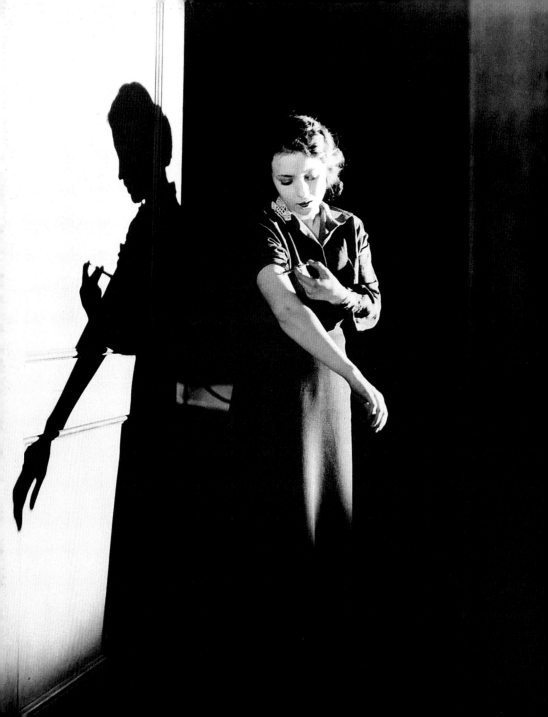

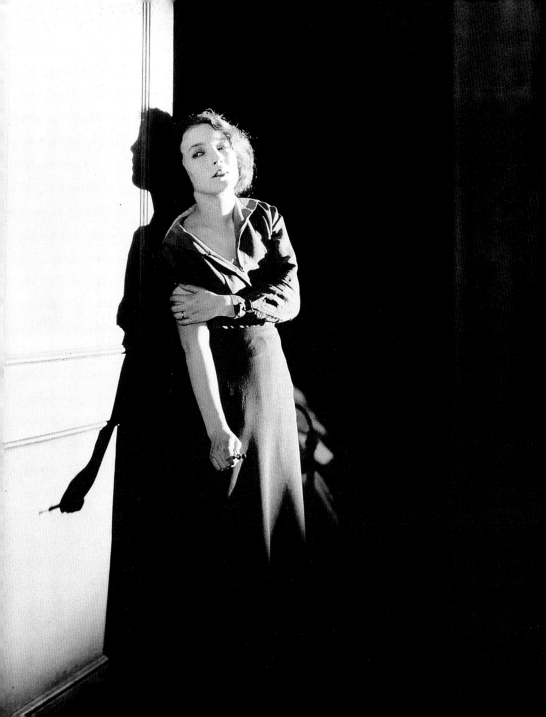

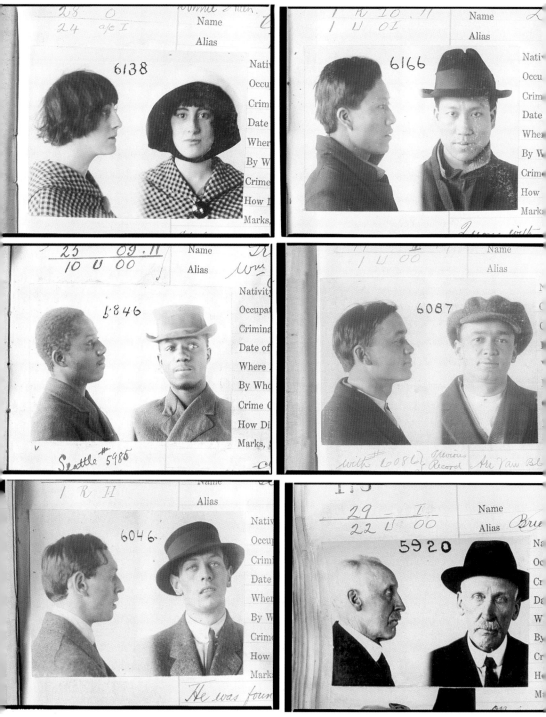

28   0
24   a/c I

Name
Alias

6138

Nativ
Occu
Crim
Date
Wher
By W
Crime
How I
Marks,

---

1   R   IO   II
1   U   OI

Name
Alias

6166

Nati
Occu
Crim
Date
Wher
By W
Crim
How
Marks

---

23   09   II
10   U   00

Name
Alias   Wm

5846

Nativity
Occupat
Crimina
Date of
Where
By Who
Crime C
How Di
Marks,

Seattle # 5985

---

1   U   00

Name
Alias

6087

Nativit
Occu
Crim
Date
Wher
By Wh
Crime
How
Marks

with # 6087   Previous Record   An Van B6

---

1   R   II

Name
Alias

6046

Nativ
Occu
Crim
Date
Wher
By W
Crime
How
Marks

He was foun

---

29   I
22   U   00

Name
Alias   Bru

5920

Na
Oc
Cr
Da
W
By
Cr
H
M

Opiomania

There was Morphine Sue and the Poppy Face Kid,
Climbed up snow ladders and down they skid.—Anonymous

*O*n 10 August 1916, twenty-one-year-old Connie Snyder, alias Connie McDermott, alias Mrs. Dutch Snyder, was picked up by Vancouver police for possession of narcotics, a relatively new and haphazardly enforced offence in North America. Women, up to this time, were thought to be more prone to addiction than men—in surveys of American communities between 1880 and 1913, women comprised some 60 to 70 per cent of opium and morphine users—yet, in 1916, Miss Snyder was one of only nineteen women held on narcotics charges out of over five hundred such arrests.[1]

Morphine use by women was declining, in part because of improvements to health and sanitation and in part because of the introduction of laws controlling narcotics. Most women addicts received their narcotics from doctors and pharmacists, but as the laws tightened, the medical profession dispensed drugs far less casually. As these legal sources for narcotics dried up, the number of women addicts fell, but the rate of addiction among men grew.[2]

Twentieth-century changes to drug laws continued the trend established during the previous century, when pharmaceutical laws were tightened in an effort to control sales of all drugs. In addition, through the late 1800s and early 1900s, the United States and Australia restricted importations of opium for smoking but overlooked medical opium. By the late nineteenth century, as temperance movements cried out against intoxication and anti-opium leagues lobbied for a halt to the opium trade, critics turned their attention to medical opium, especially opium-laced patent medicines.

Patent medicines came under fire largely because of their mysterious compositions. In 1906 in Britain and the United States, and in 1908 in Canada, laws requiring disclosure of ingredients and limitation of narcotic content were instituted. Then, within the next decade, tough antinarcotic laws—Britain's Dangerous Drugs Act (1920), France's *Loi des stupéfiants* (1916) and the United States' Harrison Narcotic Act (1914)—were passed, controlling medicinal opium, morphine, heroin and cocaine. The Harrison Act required pharmacists and doctors to register with the Department of the Treasury, pay taxes and keep records of narcotics prescribed or dispensed. The purpose of the act was not to penalize drug users but to create a "revenue and control measure."[4] Its wording was open to interpretation, however, and the result was a far tighter control than originally intended.

While individual countries were busy passing their own laws, the international community was meeting about what was seen as a worldwide crisis in opium traffic. At the First International Opium Conference of 1909 in Shanghai and the Second and Third Conferences of 1912 and 1914 in The Hague, directions in opium control were discussed. Not all countries attended, nor were all attending countries prepared to completely adhere to the conferences' conclusions, notably opium-producing Greece, Serbia and Turkey. But there was a general determination to work towards the control of the production and distribution of opium and its derivatives.

Bingham Dai "The person under the influence of opium is enjoying a moral holiday."[3]

La Guerre des stupéfiants, cover for an issue of *Police magazine,* featuring a melodramatic article on the thriving drug trade by Jean Créteuil. Photo uncredited. 2 October 1938.

1 fr. 50

POLICE MAGAZINE

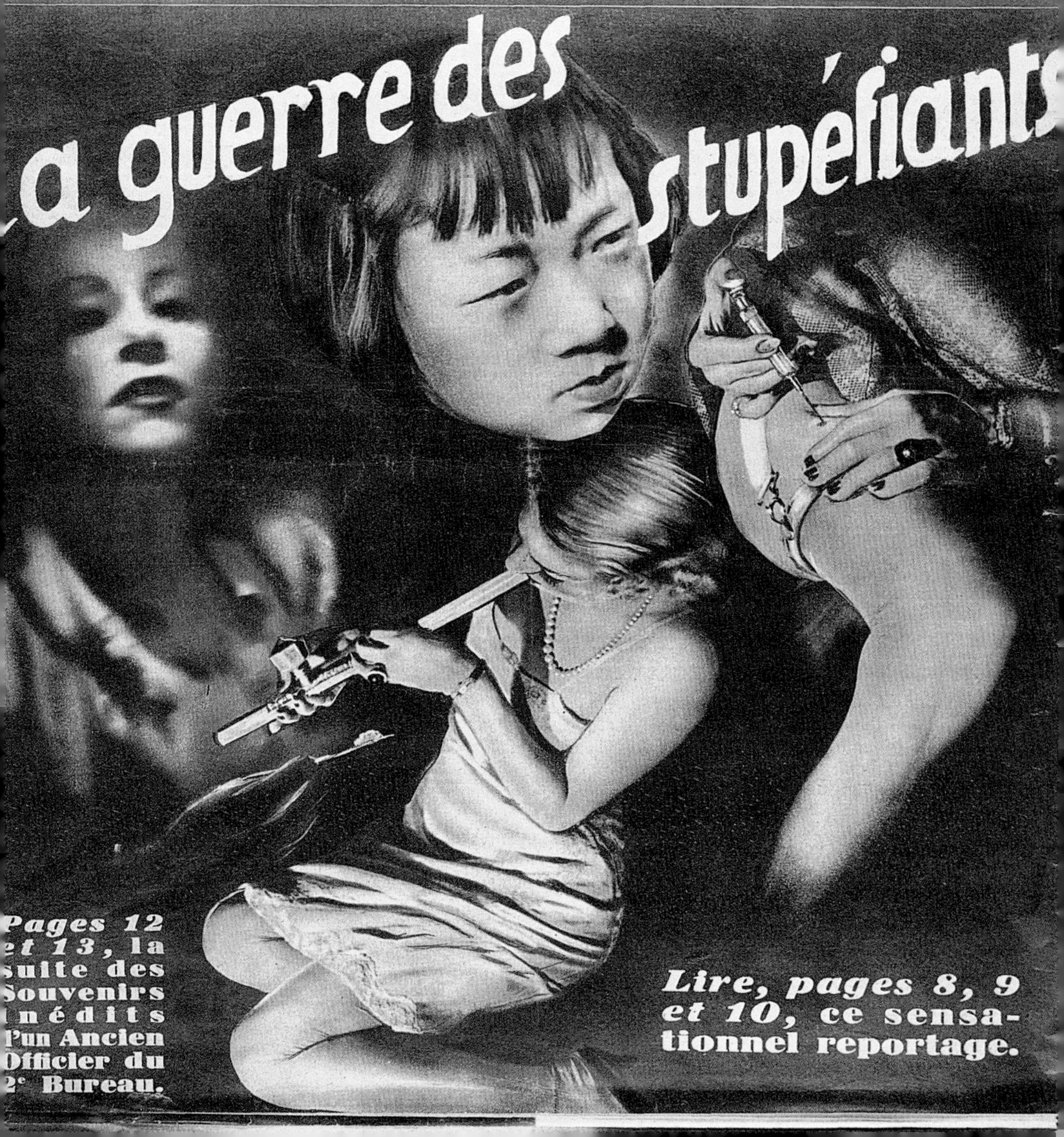

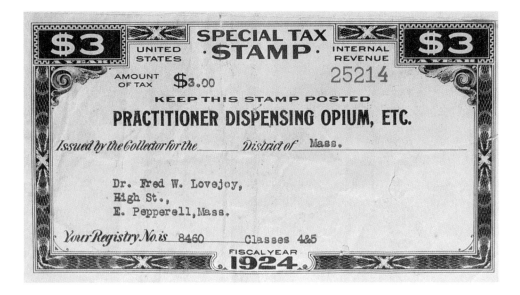

United States Narcotics Stamp Tax, 1924. The first law regulating drugs in the United States was the Boylan Bill of 1911, which limited access to hypodermic needles, followed by the Harrison Narcotics Act of 1914, which restricted the sale and administration of narcotics.

The effect of legislation against narcotics had three visible results; the first was increased drug costs, which, in turn, led to an increase in petty crime. Violet McNeal, a morphine-addicted quack medicine peddler, noted that a dram of morphine, which could be had for 60¢ before the Harrison Act, cost $35.00 after.[5] The second, more traumatic effect, was to make a heretofore legal activity illegal. Suddenly drug addicts who had been cared for or pitied or simply ignored were now criminals, liable to be thrown in jail for what had previously been considered a moral weakness. The third result was the appearance of an even newer kind of criminal, the narcotics dealer.

The medical profession was no longer the principal originator of addiction. In a study done by Kolb and Du Mez in 1924, of ten thousand New York addicts questioned only 2 per cent could fault their doctors for their condition. Increasingly, addiction was being linked to association with other addicts.[7]

Although some physicians and clinics continued to try to cure drug dependencies medically, addicts were now largely considered to be degenerates or criminals. And yet, perversely, popular culture—through movies, magazines, novels—glamourized addicts, whose lifestyles offered excitement mixed with a touch of danger. Crime organizations took over the cultivation, manufacture and distribution of opium and its derivatives, turning an erstwhile legitimate and thriving business into a phenomenally powerful industry that no government could eradicate, let alone control.

Throughout the late 1800s and into the early years of the twentieth century, most opium imagery concentrated on either simple observations of drug use habits or the dreamy worlds of the user. Only occasionally would an artist attempt to show the despair of a poor wretch locked in morphine's grip. With criminalization, the depictions of drug use changed. Fevered by the excitement of capturing this now-reprehensible behaviour, artists and photographers in the early twentieth century played up the dangers, desperation and sordidness of opium and morphine addiction. Book and magazine covers breathlessly intertwined drugs and violence, drugs and sex, drugs and youth or all of them on the same action-packed cover. Women adorned these covers, sometimes as victims of drug pushers, sometimes as perpetrators of vice. *Teen-Age Gangs*, *Le Morphinomane assassin*, *Counterfeit Wife (Gin et laudanum)*, *Dope, Inc.*, *Junkie*, *Narcotic Agent*, *The Dream Peddlers*, *The Needle* and *Marijuana Murders* are only a few of the titles that appeared between 1910 and 1960.

Counterfeit Wife, 1947

"Come around some time, big boy, and bring your laudanum."

"What's the matter with tonight?"

—Gerta Dawson and Mike Shayne[6]

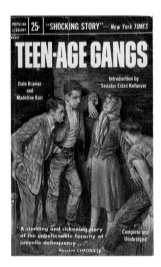

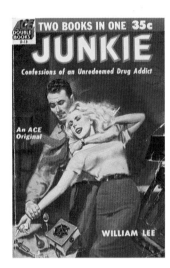

Clockwise from top left: Teen-Age Gangs by Dale Kramer and Madeline Karr delivered a heated diatribe against the antisocial behaviour of youth. And, of course, drugs—marijuana, heroin and morphine—were at the heart of the problem. Uncredited cover art. Popular Library, 1954.
Junkie by William Lee (William Burroughs). Its ambivalent message is tempered by the co-publication—in the same volume—of the anti-drug story *Narcotic Agent* by Maurice Helbrant (*facing page*). Ace Books, 1953. Courtesy Reg Daggit
Le Morphinomane assassin by Réginald Harlowe. Detective Raoul Péterson infiltrates a drug ring in order to discover which of four morphinomaniacs killed pharmacist Henri Durieu. Uncredited cover art. Les éditions Harlowe, c. 1950.
Le Drageoir d'opium by A. Samson. Set in the late 1700s, this is an absurd tale about a young noblewoman who elopes with a stranger. Opium bonbons, given to her father as compensation, turn him into a jaundiced, raving maniac. Cover by P. H. Lafon. Flachon, c. 1920.

Morphine in Belgium "There is no city more willing than cosmopolitan Antwerp to go along with debauchery, lust or drug taking, three vices which breed all the ills that humanity suffers."—*Le morphinomane assassin*[8]

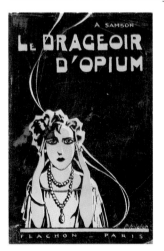

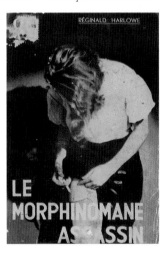

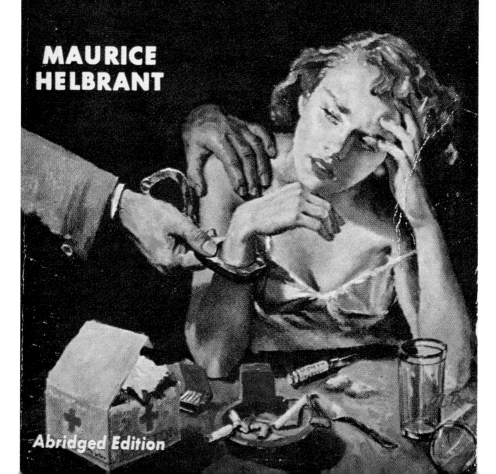

TWO BOOKS IN ONE 35c

Gripping True Adventures of a
T-Man's War Against the Dope Menace

NARCOTIC AGENT

MAURICE HELBRANT

Abridged Edition

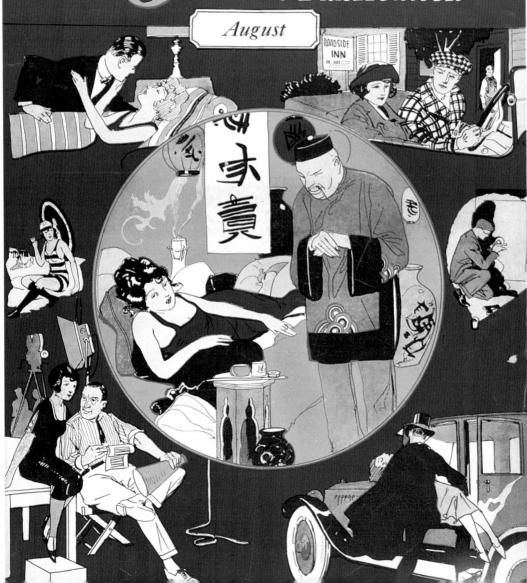

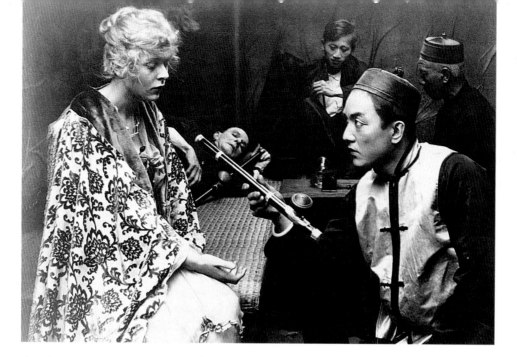

Above: *The Secret Sin*, US 1915. Blanche Sweet plays Grace, who falls ill after visiting an opium den. She becomes addicted to drugs when her doctor prescribes morphine. Sweet also had roles in other drug-related movies: *For His Son*, 1912, and *Public Opinion*, 1916. Courtesy the Library of Congress

Facing page: *True Confessions*. The lead article of this inaugural issue, "Experiences of a Dope Slave," by Babe Lamont, covers everything—cocaine, morphine, heroin—but not the opium smoking shown on the cover. Uncredited. August 1922.

These scandalous images transferred perfectly to the big screen. Scenes showing depraved white women lolling about in dark and evil Chinese opium dens were dream situations for film. A surprising number of movies picturing opium smoking were made until the 1930s in studios in the United States, France and Britain. *Chinese Opium Den*, 1894; *Rube in an Opium Joint*, 1905; *Le Rêve d'un fumeur d'opium*, 1908; *The Secret Sin*, 1915, are but a few.*

Many of the early films used opium more for its pictorial, exotic appeal than as a moral lesson. Some, such as Charlie Chaplin's *Easy Street* (1917), are downright hilarious. In this movie, Chaplin, a bumbling policeman, gets the extra kick he needs to capture a brute by accidentally sitting down on a hop-head's hypodermic needle. Another drug comedy, possibly the

* A more extensive listing can be found in the Appendix.

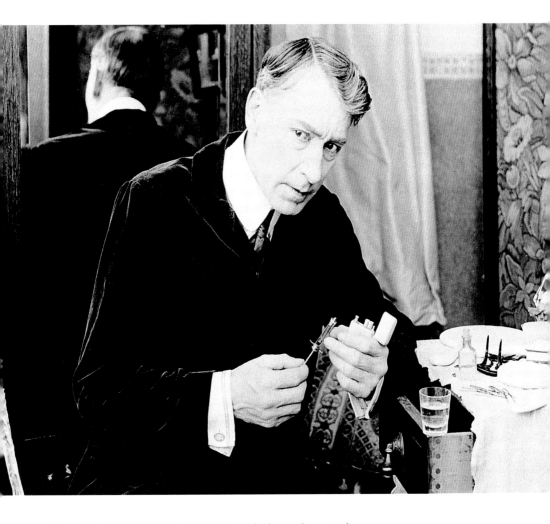

The Devil's Needle, US 1916. Artist's model Renée (Norma Talmadge) introduces artist John Minton (Tully Marshall, shown here) to drugs. He tries them reluctantly but finds that they improve his concentration and becomes hopelessly addicted. Courtesy BFI Stills, Posters and Designs

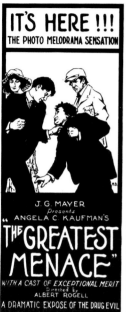

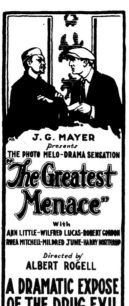

The Greatest Menace, US 1923, released one month before Human Wreckage, is a now-lost film about the son of a D.A. who becomes addicted to drugs while writing about the realities of life. When arrested for a drug-related murder, he is successfully defended by his lawyer sister and goes straight. Starring Robert Gordon and Ann Little. Courtesy the Library of Congress

Promotional propaganda for The Greatest Menace suggested enlisting shops to join in cooperative advertising. Sample wording for a clothing shop: "The Greatest Menace in life can easily be avoided by wearing a collar that will not saw your head off every time it is worn."

zaniest movie ever made, is *The Mystery of the Leaping Fish* (1916), starring Bessie Love as the fish-blower girl and Douglas Fairbanks as the narcotics-powered detective Coke Ennyday, who is hired to round up a band of opium smugglers.

By the 1920s, however, movies with drug themes were firmly moralistic, vilifying drug society while somehow managing to glorify it. Because morphine didn't have the same exotic appeal as opium smoking, filmmakers searched for another enticing element and found the youth angle, to great success. In movies such as *The Pace that Kills* (1928) and *Narcotic* (1933), innocent kids are introduced to "dope," either as a headache powder or as harmless party fun. They fall for the drug in a big way, and soon opium, morphine, cocaine and heroin take over their lives. One could go see any of a number of these heart-wrenching antidrug movies, including *The Devil's Needle*, *The Drug Terror* and *The Greatest Menace*. It's doubtful that these productions convinced any but God-fearing citizens to stay away from drugs, but they did succeed in magnifying the problem beyond reality.

In real-life Hollywood, the stories of the silent-screen stars who reputedly used drugs without restraint captivated the public.

Magazines were filled with gossip about sultry vamp Barbara La Marr, who had a preference for the finest Benares opium; dashing director William Desmond Taylor, murdered in mysterious circumstances, involving a love foursome and narcotics; and Alma Rubens, a morphine addict who tried to stab an ambulance attendant. The careers of many of these people were ruined by drugs, but Wallace Reid's, in particular, came to an abrupt and nasty end when his addiction to morphine, compounded by a heavy dependence on alcohol, left him unable to work. It is reported that during the filming of one of his last pictures, he had to be propped up in front of the camera. In 1922, Reid's wife, actress Dorothy Davenport, committed the actor to a sanitarium for a morphine cure and he never reemerged. After his death, she produced the now-lost antidrug film *Human Wreckage*.[11]

Narcotics in Hollywood is a complete story unto itself, and it finds parallels with the world of stage and music, all of which received unprecedented attention from magazines and newspapers; reading them now, one gets the impression that the world had succumbed to an epidemic of addiction.

In spite of, or perhaps because of, the evidence of misery, corruption and waste, our fascination with opium persists to this day. Stereotype-shattering contradictions such as the ease with which strict Victorians accommodated drug habitués throw into question our notions of pre-twentieth century lives, habits and values and, in doing so, help clarify our present-day attitudes towards drugs and drug addiction. And though we may try to shake off the myth of the Morphean slumber and the promise of profound dreams and boundless creativity, it's doubtful that opium will ever let us.

Clockwise from top left:
Mabel Normand (1894–1930) was a leading silent-screen comedienne. Her behaviour was food for the gossip columnists and rumours started that she was addicted to drugs. Uncredited photo.

Barbara La Marr (1896–1926), known as the "girl who was too beautiful," died of a narcotics overdose. She starred in such films as *Arabian Love,* 1922, and *The Prisoner of Zenda,* 1922. Uncredited photo.

Alma Rubens (1897–1931) starred in a number of films, including *Intolerance,* 1916. In spite of time spent in sanatoriums, her attempts to overcome her addiction were futile. In 1931, she was arrested at the California/Mexico border for possession of morphine.[9] Uncredited photo, from "Studio News and Gossip East and West," *Photoplay,* March 1925, 57.

Wallace Reid (1891–1923) was said to have hung out with the "Hollywood Hell-Raisers," a group devoted to a "life of drink, dope and debauchery."[10] Photo by Evans, from "The Real Wally" by Dorothy Davenport Reid, *Photoplay,* March 1925, 59.

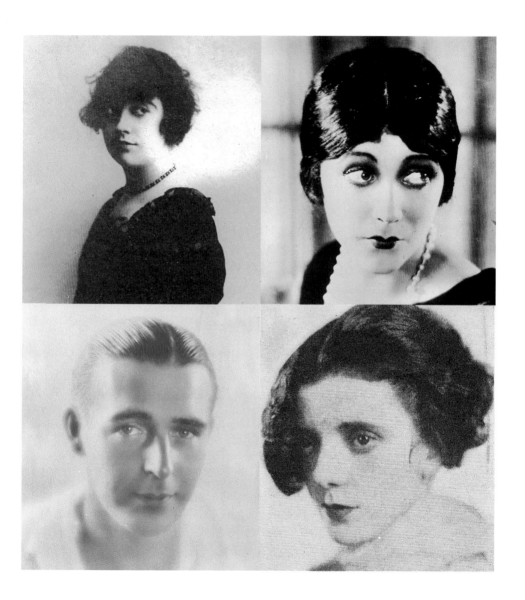

1906); Dr. H. H. Kane (US 1880s); Dr. J.C. Hoffman Cure (US 1906); Dr. J. Edward Allport System (US 1906);

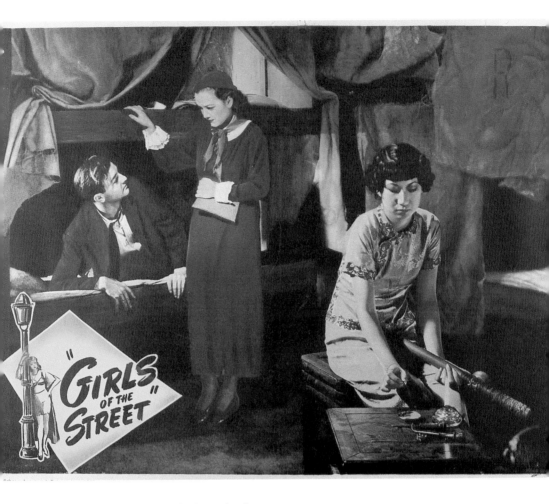

Girls of the Street aka *Cocaine Fiends* aka *The Pace that Kills,* US 1937, starring Dean Benton, Lois January, Lois Lindsay, Noel Madison, Sheila Manners and Edward Phillips. A remake of the 1928 silent film *The Pace that Kills,* this film is about good kids who come to the city and fall prey to the lure of fast living. Although cocaine is highlighted in one of the alternative titles to this film and is the drug that starts the downward slide, morphine, heroin, marijuana and opium smoking, as shown in this lobby card, all play a part in this film of abject hopelessness.

Appendix

Lack of space prevents the inclusion of television shows, narcotics-smuggling movies such as *The French Connection* and teen marijuana flicks such as *Reefer Madness*. The following films either feature or include a scene with laudanum, morphine or opium smoking. Where the particular drug is clear from the title, I have omitted specifying it.

Ahen senso (The Opium War), Japan 1943

Ann Vickers, US 1933, cocaine

Baby Doll, US 1956, paregoric

Bite the Bullet, US 1976, laudanum

Bits of Life, US 1921, opium smoking

Black Fear, US 1915 (1916?), narcotics

The Bondwomen, US 1915, narcotics

Broken Blossoms aka *The Chink and the Child, Scarlet Blossoms, Yellow Man and the Girl*, US 1919, opium smoking

Case of a Doped Actress, GB 1919, narcotics

Charlie Chan in Shanghai, US 1935, opium smuggling

Chinese Opium Den, US 1894

A Chinese Opium Joint, US 1898

Cocaine Fiends aka *The Pace that Kills, The Girls of the Street*, US 1937, narcotics, opium smoking

Confessions of an Opium Eater aka *Evils of Chinatown*, US 1962, opium smoking

Il Conformista (The Conformist), Italy 1969, morphine

The Derelict, US 1914, narcotics

The Devil's Assistant, US 1914, narcotics

The Devil's Needle aka *The Dope Fiend, Drugged Hopes, The White Curse*, US 1916, narcotics

The Devil's Profession, GB 1916, narcotics

The Dividend, US 1916, narcotics

Doctor from Seven Dials aka *Corridors of Blood*, GB 1958, narcotics

Dope, US 1914

Drifting, US 1923, opium smuggling

The Drug Terror aka *The Underworld Exposé, The Cocaine Traffic*, US 1914

The Drug Traffic, US 1914 (remade 1923)

Easy Street, US 1917, narcotics

Farewell My Concubine, HK/China 1993, opium smoking

For His Son, US 1912, narcotics

Frailty, GB 1921, morphine

Gothic, GB 1986, laudanum

The Greatest Menace, US 1923, narcotics

Great Hero of China, China 1993, kung fu and opium

A Hatful of Rain, US 1957, narcotics

Hei lu (Deadly China Doll, The Opium Trail), HK 1972, opium smuggling

Heroes for Sale, US 1933, narcotics

Hollywood Cavalcade, US 1939, opium smoking

Human Wreckage, US 1923, morphine

Indochine, France 1992, opium smoking

Interview with a Vampire, US 1994, laudanum

Intrigue, US 1947, narcotics smuggling

Kansas City, US 1996, laudanum

Kri Kri fuma oppio (Boomer Smokes Opium), Italy 1913

Lady Sings the Blues, US 1972, narcotics

The Last Emperor, Italy/HK/GB 1984, opium smoking

The Letter, US 1940, opium smoking

Lightning Fists of Shaolin aka *Opium and the Kung Fu Master*, HK 1984

Lightning Raider, US 1919, opium smoking

Lin zexu (The Opium War), China 1959

Long Day's Journey into Night, US 1962, morphine

McCabe and Mrs. Miller, US 1976, opium smoking

The Man Who Came Back, US 1924 (remade 1931), opium smoking

The Man with the Golden Arm, US 1956, morphine

Mask of Fu Manchu, US 1932, opium smoking

Monkey on My Back, US 1957, morphine

Morfinisten (The Morphine Takers, Slaves of Morphine), Denmark 1911

My Life and Times with Antonin Artaud, France 1993, narcotics

The Mystery of Edwin Drood, US 1935, opium smoking

The Mystery of the Leaping Fish, US 1916, narcotics

Naked Lunch, Canada 1991, narcotics

Narcotic, US 1933

Narcotic Spectre, US 1914

The Narcotic Story, US 1956, heroin

Once Upon a Time in America, US 1984, opium smoking

Opium, Germany 1919

The Opium Connection aka *The Poppy Is Also a Flower*, US 1966, opium smuggling

Opiumsdrømmen (Opium Dreams), Denmark 1914

The Opium Smugglers, US 1912

The Pace that Kills, US 1928, narcotics

Pandaemonium, GB 2000, laudanum

Pied Piper Malone, US 1924, opium smoking

Public Opinion, US 1916, narcotics

Razzia sur la chnouf, France 1955, narcotics smuggling

The Red Kimono, US 1925, heroin

The Red Violin, Canada 1998, opium smoking

Le Rêve d'un fumeur d'opium (Dream of an Opium Fiend), France 1908

The Rise of Susan aka *Cosette*, US 1916, narcotics

The Road to Ruin, US 1934, narcotics

A Romance of the Underworld, US 1918, narcotics

Rube in an Opium Joint, US 1905, opium smoking

Queen X, US 1914, opium smoking

Satan Opium, Germany 1914 or 1915

The Secret Sin, US 1915, opium smoking

Shanghai Surprise, GB 1986, opium smuggling

Sherlock Holmes und das Halsband des Todes (Sherlock Holmes and the Deadly Necklace), Germany/Italy/France 1962, opium smoking

Sowing the Wind, US 1921, opium smoking

Die Spinnen (The Spiders), Germany 1919, opium smoking

Tian Di, China 1994, opium smuggling

Tian luo di wang (Gunmen), China 1988, opium trade

Tombstone, US 1993, laudanum, opium smoking

Tong Man, US 1919, opium smuggling

To the Ends of the Earth, US 1948, opium smuggling

The Vortex, GB 1928, narcotics

The Whispering Chorus, US 1918, opium

The Wings of the Dove, GB 1997, opium smoking

Xiang yi yu tiao zhan (Challenge to Devil Area), China 1991, opium trade

Yapian zhanzheng (The Opium War), China 1997

Yellow Claw, GB 1920, opium smoking

Notes

Introduction, pp. 1–15

Quote from Ovid, *Metamorphoses*, Book XI, 317.

Quote from Cocteau, *Opium: Diary of a Cure*, 86.

Quoted in Day, 235.

1 Smith, 165–66.
2 Squire, 1342–61.
3 De Quincey, 1907 (1821), 177–78.
4 Cobbe, 44.
5 Quoted in Day, 234.
6 "The Mayor and the Tenements," 699.
7 Saussay, 171.
8 Browning, vol. II, 126; De Quincey, 1907 (1821), 181.
9 Hasselquist, 176.
10 Chardin, 244.
11 "Opium." In *Encyclopædia Britannica*, vol. XVII, 811.

The Search for Health, pp. 17–43

Quote from Molière: *The Imaginary Invalid*, adapted by Miles Malleson, Act III, 68.

Quote from Lindesmith, 159.

Quote from Cobbe, 29.

Quote from Psalmanazar, 48.

1 Richard Morton, cited in Legouis, 298.
2 Pliny, 275–76.
3 Kritikos, 19–20.
4 Gunther, 456–60.
5 Pliny, notes, 300; Sydenham, "Epistolary Dissertation," 105.
6 Wootton, vol. I, 289; Watson, 3, 37; Pliny 300; Wootton, vol. II, 40.
7 Levey, 4; Wootton, vol. I, 110; Levey, formulas throughout.

8 Sydenham, "Epistolary Dissertation," 85; "Processus Integri," 236, 248, 257, 263, 266, 268, 275, 300; Darwin, *Zoonomia*, vol. II, 64, 99, 131, 138, 276.
9 Molière, 650 and footnote; Raynaud, 421.
10 Piozzi, 125.
11 Fracastoro, 199.
12 Cowen, 46, 56, 52; Trease, 42–46.
13 Trease, 84; Cowen, 68.
14 Pachter, 136; Paracelsus, 169.
15 Bacon, 149; Sydenham, "Epistolary Dissertation," 98.
16 Packard, 270; Maehle, 132–33.
17 Cowen, 91; *Pharmacopœia Londinensis*, 1–3, 40, 41.
18 Calkins, 141.
19 Pomet, 218.
20 Jones, 8.
21 Bacon, 150; Browne, vol. I, 275, vol. III, 24–25.
22 Maehle, 136–37; Cowen, 102; Maehle, 146.
23 Summerson, 32.
24 Garth, 4.
25 Seaman, 18.
26 Jones, 8.
27 Cowen, 95; Porter, 263; Morgagni, 5.
28 Darwin, vol. II, 43–44.
29 Maehle, 172–73.
30 King-Hele, 83, 121; Darwin's quote reported by Wedgwood in *Letters of Josiah Wedgwood*, vol. II, 541–52, quoted in King-Hele, 131–32.
31 King-Hele, 247.
32 Ibid., 13.
33 Young, 1753, 31, 34.

34 Young, 1753, 6–7.
35 Young, 1753, 68; Foreman, 108; Young, 1753, 63, 73.
36 Calkins, 185.
37 De Quincey, 1907 (1821), 179.
38 Csáth, 104.
39 Cobbe, 301.
40 Ibid., 161.
41 De Quincey, 1907 (1821), 21.
42 "Opium and Alcohol Compared," quoted in Day, 209.
43 De Quincey, 1907 (1821), 2, 7.
44 Blair, 47–57.
45 Day, 12.
46 Cobbe, 27–28.
47 Tailhade, 1914, 270.
effects spread: Lindesmith, 22–24, 28, 47; Cobbe, 34–36, 47–49, 53, 62, 64–66, 70, 75, 78, 80, 86, 92–94, 97, 101, 104, 106, 159, 194–97, 204, 218–26, 228, 233, 239, 242–43, 262, 314; Blair, throughout; De Quincey, 1907 (1821), 192, 193; Calkins, 70, 71, 81.

Drink Me, pp. 45–77

Quote from Browning, vol. I, letter to Mitford, February 1840, 178.

Quote from Collins, 1866, Part 2, 145.

Quote from Browning, vol. II, letter to Mitford, December 1842, 126.

1 Quoted in Pachter, 137; Pagel, 330; Paracelsus, 179.
2 *Pharmacopœia Londinensis*, 56; LaWall, 312, 420; according to Wootton, vol. II, 145, Black Drop was made from opium, verjuice (juice of wild crab), nutmeg, saffron and yeast.

3 Sydenham, "Schedula Monitoria III," 221–23, 236, 237; LaWall, 280.
4 Sydenham, "Epistolary Dissertation," 85, 88, 103; Sydenham, "Epistolary Dissertation," 108; "Processus Integri," 284.
5 Collins, 1994 (1862), 451; Trease, 179.
6 Jardillier, 171; Wootton writes that Rousseau's Laudanum was also fermented, vol. II, 144; 9 LaWall, 420–21.
7 De Quincey, 1907 (1821), 209; Collins, 1994 (1862), 407; Caine, 1908, 339; Cobbe, 58; Stoker, 137; Alcott, 165, 190.
8 "A 'Laudanum' District," 311.
9 Hibbert, 1972, 248–50, 171.
10 "The Narcotics We Indulge In," 612; Calkins, 36; Lindesmith, 185.
11 Hibbert, 1972, 75–76, 81, 248–50; 1997, 258, 280.
12 Foreman, 86, 168, 299, 369, 130.
13 "The Maniac" was first published in *The Oracle* in September 1791, as "Insanity," Levey, 165; Molloy, 218.
14 Bernhardt, 322, 324.
15 Pollock, 78–9; Milner cited in Pollock, 80; Pollock, 278.
16 Randolph, quoted in Garland, 371.
17 Martineau, 146.
18 Pichois, 98; Dorsenne, 40.
19 Cobbe, 177.
20 Hayter, 1968, 331, 334–35.
21 Kunitz et al., 838–39; Calkins, 70.
22 Rousseau, 111, 181.
23 Manna was the dried sap of European ash used as both a laxative and a balm; Steegmuller, 224, 219, 206; Galiani, 424, 533.
24 Alcott, 191; Brontë, 1992 (1848), 181; Collins, 1886, Pt. I, 270; Pt. II, 146.
25 Borgman, 99; Boswell, 1271; Crabbe, 161.
26 Gosse, 11–12, 287–90; quoted in Gosse, 90.
27 Boswell, 1271.
28 Gosse, 287–90.
29 Buchan, 168, 169, 177, 179; quoted in Buchan, 193.
30 Buchan, 169.

31 Quoted in Cottle, 453, 459, 464.
32 Cottle, 385.
33 De Quincey, 1907 (1821), 9; Lucas, 55; Lefebure, 30, 35; De Quincey, 1889, 167; Holmes, 37, 40, 46; Hayter, 1968, 216; Cottle, 367, 388, 373.
34 Cottle, 416, 419, 421; Hayter, 1968, 80.
35 Lefebure, 178–79; Wordsworth, 33, 35, 101, 172n.
36 De Quincey, 1907 (1821), 225–26.
37 Ibid., 15, 196, 189.
38 Lindop thoroughly examines De Quincey's penury and his repeated efforts to free himself from opium; Cobbe, 183, 12.
39 Allem, 28.
40 Balzac, 814; Bory, 126, 151.
41 Quoted in Moore, 1901 (1829), 113.
42 Grosskurth, 64; Moore, 1901 (1829), 69; Elwin, 340; Quoted in Elwin, 413; Elwin, 347; Moore, 1901 (1829), 478.
43 Dunn, 61, 149; Dowden, 242.
44 Shelley, 164.
45 Byron, 4; Keats, "The Eve of St. Agnes," verse 27, "Ode to a Nightingale," lines 1–3, 202, 207.
46 Brown, 62–64, 69, 89; Bate, 686–87.
47 Thackeray, vol. II, 21.
48 Fletcher, 45–46; quoted in Fletcher, 45.
49 Mudge, 36.
50 Coleridge, Sara, *Pretty Lessons*.
51 J. Tennent, 1734, quoted in Lewis, 324.
52 "Opium-Eating," 431.
53 Calkins, 286.
54 Coleridge, 452; Mudge, 147.
55 Martineau, 146, 470 (Martineau's parentheses), 473.
56 Browning, vol. I, 337; Hayter, 1962, 65.
57 Moore, 1997, 150, 214.
58 Peters, 148–50; Winter, 211; Peters, 407; Sir William Ferguson cited in Peters, 336; Winter, 212; Peters, 240.
59 Caine, 1908, 340; Winter, 213; Caine, 1908, 340; Collins, 1994 (1862), intro by Ford, xiv–xv.
60 Wilson 303; Walsh, 61.
61 Walsh, 22, 60; Hayter, 1968, 273.

62 Collins, 1866, Pt. II, 146.
63 Collins, 1946 (1868), 371.
64 Collins, 1866, Pt. I, 158.
65 Alcott, 191.
66 Quote from Hammett, 1965 (1929), 55.
67 Galdós, 532–33.
68 Gaskell, vol. II, 247; vol. I, 264, 268.
69 Calkins, 96.
70 Stoker, 134–35.
71 Cobbe, 75; Calkins, 46.
72 "Coroners' Inquests," 239, 303; "Suicide of Mr. Isaac Cohen," 205; "Epitome of News," 381; this kind of rhubarb was used as a laxative; "Accidental Poisoning," 529.
73 "An Indianapolis woman . . . ," 415.
74 Rabbe, 119.
75 Hunt, 297–305; Caine, 1882, 15.
76 From Victor Hugo, *Chants du crépuscule*, quoted in Yvorel, 32–33; Liederkerke, 21; Yvorel, 34.
77 Holoman, 60, 47, 100, 572.
78 Sand, 194–95.
79 Orieux, 485–90.
80 Stendhal, 380–84.
81 Eliot, 672–80; "Death From Drinking Laudanum and Brandy," 209.
82 Collins, 1994 (1862), 407, 614n.
83 Stowe, 250.
84 De Quincey, 1862, 106–9.
85 Thackeray, vol. III, 319.
86 Stowe, 364.

The Possessed, pp. 79–101

Quote from Guaita, 90.
Quote from Dorsenne, 18.
Quote from Alphonse Daudet, *L'Évangeliste*, 245, Daudet's ellipses.
Quote from Dr. Zambaco, quoted in Sharkey, 64.
1 The date of the experiment is reported variously as 1804 or 1805; the results were published in 1805 and 1817, Weill, 8; Sertürner, cited in Maehle, 193.
2 Weill, 8; Maehle, 191–92; Bachmann and Coppel, 99.
3 Derosne, 258–59; Maehle, 190; Derosne, still influenced by the

revolution, the journal date is 30 Nivôse, an XI; Maehle, 191; Séguin had been thrown in jail in the intervening years for allegedly misappropriating public funds, Bachmann and Coppel, 98; Séguin, 225–47.

4 Young, 1992, 142; Wooton, vol. II, 68; Boyle, quoted in Summerson, 32.

5 Nightingale, quoted in Cook, 106.

6 McGrew, 17, 98; Goldsmith, 108; Nightingale, quoted in Cook, 106; Pickering, 173–74.

7 Bosc de Veze, 55–56.

8 Louis Faucher, *Contribution à l'étude du rêve morphinique et de morphinomanie*, thesis, 1910–11, quoted in Lindesmith, 25.

9 Verne, 184.

10 Pavel, 6, 72–73; Heine, "Morphine," lines 9–10, 806–7.

11 Daudet, 1925, 30; 1915, 230–31.

12 Wallace, 21, 22.

13 Cocteau, 1957 (1930), 21.

14 Jullian, 13; Lorrain, cited in Jullian, 44.

15 Tailhade, 1914, 268; Liedekerke, 236–37; Bachmann and Coppel, 126.

16 Liedekerke, 220; Pia, 11.

17 Jullian, 78.

18 Quoted in Cocteau, 1956, 141.

19 Francis and Gontier, vol. I, 188–89, 223; Lorenz, 54, 95.

20 Liedekerke 259; Thurman, 77; Quella-Villéger, 129; Francis and Gontier, vol. II, 128.

21 Pickering, 233; Proust, refs. to Trional and Veronal, throughout, to heroin, 205; Hayman, 212, 331, 477.

22 Tailhade, 1914, 269; Liedekerke, 15; Lerner, 189; Tuchman, 92.

23 Tailhade, 1907, 21.

24 Tailhade, 1907, 21; Daudet, 1925, 26; Liedekerke, 246; Quella-Villéger, 129; Lemaitre, 207; Francis and Gontier, vol. I, 195, 280; Thurman, 401–5.

25 James, diary entry date 4 December 1891, 244.

26 Sterne, 190, 199, 232.

27 James, 75, 77, 78, 60.

28 Sheaffer, 21–22.

29 O'Neill, 120.

30 Quoted in Anthony, 138.

31 Ibid., 130, 134.

32 Huxley, 158.

33 San Francisco *Examiner*, 23 February 1908, reprinted in Palmer and Horowitz, 72.

34 Sinclair, 317.

35 Cocteau, 1957, 73.

36 Daudet, 1935 (1907), 45.

37 Jennings, 62.

38 Daudet, 1925, 7.

39 Dubut de Laforest, 12.

40 Csáth, 7–9, 17; Csáth, quoted in Intro., 18.

41 Thurman, 203.

42 Saussay, 239.

43 Kershaw, 248; London, 392.

44 Dumas, 1900 (1844–46), 348; 1957 (1852–55), 252–57; Tailhade, 1907, 10.

45 Motion, 188; strychnine alone according to Wilde, 78; Wilde, 86.

46 Thurman, 206, citing *Sido: Lettres à sa fille*, 1984; Francis and Gontier, 84, report that Willy asked Achille how much morphine would be safe.

I Like It! I Want It! pp. 103–21

1 *Nostrums*, 1911, 434; 1921, 101; Oleson, 137; Oliver, 37.

2 Cowen, 171, 167, 184; Wooton, vol. II, 162; Young, 1961, 3–4; Wooten, vol. II, 163.

3 Young, 1961, 13; LaWall, 416.

4 LaWall, 418; Young, 1992, 127; Parssinen, 42–43.

5 Dewhurst, in Dover, xi; Dover, 75.

6 Dover, 15.

7 Diver, 93.

8 Dr. Chase, undated pamphlet.

9 Chase, 574; Richardson, 1290–92.

10 Richardson, 1288; Hamlin, 85, 112.

11 Cobbe, 19.

12 Gaskell, 1906 (1848), 63.

13 Thackeray, 247.

14 O. Marshall, cited in Terry and Pellens, 96.

15 Yonge, 93; Thackeray, 247; Gaskell,

1906 (1848), 63.

16 Calkins, 123.

17 Young, 1992, 118; Beasley's specified that Mrs. Winslow's could be made with or without morphine; Oleson, 192; *Nostrums*, 1911, 318.

18 Squire, 842; *Nostrums*, 1921, 599.

19 *Secret Remedies*, 17–18; *Nostrums*, 1911, 335.

20 Young, 1961, 9.

21 *Nostrums*, 1911, 33.

22 Ibid., 416, 350.

23 Young, 1961, 118–19; Cowen, 181.

24 Oleson, 134; *Western Druggist*, reported in Holbrook, 153.

25 Anonymous addict, quoted in Day, 259.

26 Hammett, 1974 (1929), 158.

27 De Quincey, 1907 (1821), 200–201, 219.

28 Rowell, 26.

29 Adams, 16–18; *Nostrums* 1911, 177; Jennings, 471–72.

30 Jennings, 26, 28; Freud, 157.

31 Adams, 16.

32 Jennings, 30, 26, 10.

33 Jennings, 77; Burnett, quoted in Jennings, 80.

Opiomania, pp. 125–36

1 Courtwright, 36.

2 Cobbe, 189.

3 Dai, 21.

4 Lindesmith, 189.

5 McNeal, 242.

6 Halliday, 27.

7 Kolb and Du Mez cited in Dai, 37; Dai, 41.

8 Harlowe, 31.

9 Katz, 1002; Anger, 63, 64, 65.

10 Anger, 54.

11 Anger, 49, 54, 63–65; Katz, 679, 864, 959, 1002.

Bibliography

General Bibliography

Allem, Maurice. *Alfred de Musset*. Paris: Louis-Michaud, n.d.

Anger, Kenneth. *Hollywood Babylon*. San Francisco: Straight Arrow, 1975.

Anthony, Carl Sferrazza. *Florence Harding*. New York: Morrow, 1998.

Bachmann, Christian, and Anne Coppel. *Le dragon domestique: Deux siècles de relations étranges entre l'Occident et la drogue*. Paris: Albin Michel, 1989.

Bacon, Francis. *The Historie of Life and Death*. London, 1638.

Bate, Walter J. *John Keats*. Cambridge: Harvard Univ. Press, 1963.

Beasley, Henry. *The Druggist's General Receipt Book*. 9th ed. London: J & A Churchill, 1886.

Bernhardt, Sarah. *Memoirs of My Life*. New York: Benjamin Blom, 1968 (1st published 1913).

Borgman, Albert S. *Thomas Shadwell: His Life and Comedies*. New York: New York Univ. Press, 1928.

Bory, Jean-Louis. *Eugène Süe*. Paris: Hachette, 1962.

Bosc de Veze, Ernest. *De l'opium et de la morphine*. Paris: Bibliothèque des Curiosités, 1908.

Boswell, James. *Life of Johnson*. Ed. R. W. Chapman. London: Oxford Univ. Press, 1970 (1st published 1791).

Brown, Charles A. *Life of John Keats*. Ed. D. H. Bodurtha and W. B. Pope. London: Oxford Univ. Press, 1937.

Browne, Thomas. "Pseudodoxia Epidemica." In *The Works of Sir Thomas Browne*. Ed. C. Sayle. Vols. I and III. Edinburgh: John Grant, 1912 (1st published 1682 and 1672).

Browning, Elizabeth Barrett. *The Letters of Elizabeth Barrett Browning to Mary Russell Mitford 1836–1854*. 3 vols. Ed. E. M. B. Raymond and M. R. Sullivan. Armstrong Browning Library of Baylor Univ., Browning Inst., Wedgestone Press and Wellesley College, 1983.

Buchan, John. *Sir Walter Scott*. New York: A. L. Burt, 1932.

Caine, T. Hall. *My Story*. London: Heinemann, 1908.

———. *Recollections of Dante Gabriel Rossetti*. London: Elliot Stock, 1882.

Calkins, Alonzo. *Opium and the Opium Appetite*. Philadelphia: Lippincott, 1871.

Chardin, Jean. *Description of Persia*. 1720. Reprint, in *Sir John Chardin's Travels in Persia*. London: Argonaut, 1927 (1st published 1686).

Chase, A.W. *Dr. Chase's Recipes*. Chicago: Stanton & VanVliet, 1902.

Cobbe, William R. *Doctor Judas: A Portrayal of the Opium Habit*. Chicago: Griggs, 1895.

Cocteau, Jean. *Opium: The Diary of a Cure*. Trans. M. Crosland and S. Road. London: Peter Owen, 1957 (1st published in French, 1930).

———. *Paris Album, 1900–1914*. Trans. M. Crosland. London: W. H. Allen, 1956.

Coleridge, Edith, ed. *Memoir and Letters of Coleridge*. Vol. II. London: Henry S. King, 1873.

Cook, Sir Edward. *The Life of Florence Nightingale*. New York: Macmillan, 1942 (1st published 1913).

Cottle, Joseph. *Reminiscences of Samuel Taylor Coleridge and Robert Southey*. London: Houlston & Stoneman, 1847.

Courtwright, David T. *Dark Paradise: Opiate Addiction in America before 1940*. Cambridge: Harvard Univ. Press, 1982.

Cowen, David and William Helfand. *Pharmacy: An Illustrated History*. New York: Abrams, 1990.

Crabbe, George. *Life of the Rev. Crabbe, L.L.B.* Vol. I. London: John Murray, 1834.

Csáth, Géza. "Opium." In *The Magician's Garden and Other Stories*. Introduction M. D. Birnbaum. Trans. J. Kessler and C. Rogers. New York: Columbia Univ. Press, 1980.

Dai, Bingham. *Opium Addiction in Chicago*. Montclair, N.J.: Patterson Smith, 1970 (1st published 1937).

Darwin, Erasmus. *Zoonomia; or, The laws of organic life*. 2 vols. London, 1796.

Daudet, Léon. *Devant la douleur: Souvenirs littéraires, politiques, artistique et médicaux de 1880 à 1905*. Paris: Nouvelle Librairie Nationale, 1915.

———. *L'Homme et le poison*. Paris: Nouvelle Librairie Nationale, 1925.

Day, Horace. *The Opium Habit: with Suggestions as to the Remedy*. New York: Harper & Brothers, 1868.

De Quincey, Thomas. *Confessions of an English Opium-Eater*. London: J. M. Dent, 1907 (1st published 1821).

———. "Postscript to 'Supplementary Paper on Murder.'" In *The English Mail Coach and Other Writings*. Edinburgh: Adam & Charles Black, 1862.

———. "Samuel Taylor Coleridge." In *The Collected Writings of Thomas De Quincey*. Ed. D. Masson. Edinburgh: Adam & Charles Black, 1889 (1st published 1834–35).

Dorsenne, Jean. *La Noire idole*. Paris: La Nouvelle Revue Critique, 1930.

and his Eye Water for the Morphin Habit (US 1910); Purdy Cure (US 1906); Reliable Cure from the Opium and Morphia Hab

Dorvault, F. *Catalogue Pharmaceutique*. 2 vols. Paris: Pharmacie Centrale de France, 1877 (reprinted by Éditions du Layet, 1985).

Dover, Thomas. *The Ancient Physician's Legacy to his Country*. 2nd ed., 1742. Reprint, in *Thomas Dover's Life and Legacy*. Ed. K. Dewhurst. Metuchen, N.J.: Scarecrow, 1974 (1st published 1732).

Dowden, Edward. *The Life of Percy Bysshe Shelley*. London: Kegan Paul, Tranch, Trubner, 1926.

Dumas, Alexandre. *Mes Mémoires*. Vol. II. Paris: Gallimard, 1957 (1st published 1852–55).

Dunn, Jane. *Moon in Eclipse: A Life of Mary Shelley*. London: Weidenfeld & Nicolson, 1978.

Elwin, Malcolm. *Lord Byron's Wife*. London: Macdonald, 1962.

Fletcher, Loraine. *Charlotte Smith: A Critical Biography*. London: Macmillan, 1998.

Foreman, Amanda. *Georgiana: Duchess of Devonshire*. London: HarperCollins, 1998.

Fracastoro, Girolamo. *Fracastor: Syphilis or the French Disease*. Trans. H. Wynne-Finch. London: Heinemann Medical Books, 1935.

Francis, Claude, and Fernande Gontier. *Creating Colette: From Ingenue to Libertine, 1873–1913*. 2 vols. South Royalton, Vermont: Steerforth, 1999 (1st published in French, 1989).

Freud, Sigmund. *Cocaine Papers*. Ed. R. Byck. New York: New American Library, 1974.

Galiani, Ferdinando. *L'abbé F. Galiani, correspondance*. Ed. L. Perey and G. Maugras. Paris: Calman Lévy, 1881.

Garland, Hugh A. *The Life of John Randolph of Roanoke*. Vol. II. New York: D. Appleton, 1851.

Gaskell, Elizabeth C. *The Life of Charlotte Brontë*. 2 vols. New York: D. Appleton, 1857.

Goldsmith, Margaret. *The Trail of Opium*. London: Robert Hale, 1939.

Gosse, Philip. *Dr. Viper: The Querulous Life of Philip Thicknesse*. London: Cassell, 1952.

Grosskurth, Phyllis. *Byron: The Flawed Angel*. London: Hodder & Stoughton, 1997.

Guaita, Stanislas de. *Lettres inédites de Stanislas de Guaita au Sâr Joséphin Péladan*. Ed. Emile Dantinne. Neuchatel, Éditions Rosicruciennes, 1952.

Gunther, Robert T. *The Greek Herbal of Dioscorides*. New York: Hafner, 1959.

Hamlin, Chas. E. *Hamlin's Formulæ: Every Druggist His Own Perfumer*. Baltimore: Edward B. Read & Son, 1885.

Hasselquist, Frederik. *Voyages and Travels in the Levant in the Years 1749, 50, 51, 52*. London, 1766.

Hayman, Ronald. *Proust: A Biography*. London: Heinemann, 1990.

Hayter, Alathea. *Mrs. Browning: A Poet's Work and its Setting*. London: Faber & Faber, 1962.

———. *Opium and the Romantic Imagination*. London: Faber & Faber, 1968.

Hibbert, Christopher. *George IV: Prince of Wales 1762–1822*. New York: Harper & Row, 1972.

———. *Wellington: A Personal History*. New York: HarperCollins, 1997.

Holbrook, Stewart H. *The Golden Age of Quackery*. New York: Macmillan, 1959.

Holoman, D. Kern. *Berlioz*. Cambridge: Harvard Univ. Press, 1989.

Holmes, Richard. *Coleridge: Early Visions*. New York: Viking, 1989.

Hunt, Violet. *The Wife of Rossetti*. New York: E. P. Dutton, 1932.

James, Alice. *Alice James, her brothers—her journal*. Ed. A. Robeson Burr. New York: Dodd, Mead, 1934.

Jardillier, Marcel. *Contribution a l'étude de l'opium et des preparations opiacées du codex*. Amiens: Imprimerie Nouvelle, 1930.

Jennings, Oscar. *The Morphia Habit and its Voluntary Renunciation*. London: Bailliere, Tindall & Cox, 1909.

Jones, John. *The Mysteries of Opium Reveal'd*. London, 1700.

Jullian, Philippe. *Jean Lorrain: ou le satiricon*. Paris: Fayard, 1974 (1st published 1900).

Katz, Ephraim. *The Film Encyclopedia*. New York: Perigree, 1979.

Kershaw, Alex. *Jack London: A Life*. New York: St. Martin's, 1997.

King-Hele, Desmond. *Doctor of Revolution: The Life and Genius of Erasmus Darwin*. London: Faber & Faber, 1977.

Kunitz, Stanley J., and Vineta Colby, eds. *European Authors: 1000–1900*. New York: H. W. Wilson, 1967.

LaWall, Charles H. *Four Thousand Years of Pharmacy*. Philadelphia: J. B. Lippincott, 1927.

Lefebure, Molly. *Samuel Taylor Coleridge: A Bondage of Opium*. New York: Stein & Day, 1974.

Legouis, Pierre. *André Marvell: poète, puritain, patriot*. Paris: Henri Didier, 1928.

Lemaitre, Jules. "Ernest Renan." In *Les Contemporains, 1884 et 1885*. Paris: Société Française d'imprimerie et de librairie, c. 1903.

Lerner, Michael. *Maupassant*. New York: George Braziller, 1975.

Levey, Martin. *The Medical Formulary or Aqrābādhīn of al-Kindi*. Madison: Univ. of Wisconsin Press, 1966.

Lewis, Walter H., and M. P. F. Elvin-Lewis. *Medical Botany*. New York: John Wiley & Sons, 1977.

Liedekerke, Arnould de. *La Belle époque de l'opium*. Paris: Aux éditions de la différence, 1984.

Lindesmith, Alfred R. *Opiate Addiction*. Evanston, Illinois: Principia Press, n.d.

Lindop, Grevel. *The Opium-Eater: A Life of Thomas De Quincey*. New York: Taplinger, 1981.

Lorenz, Paul. *Sapho 1900: Renée Vivien*. Paris: Julliard, 1977.

Lucas, E. V., ed. *Charles Lamb and the Lloyds*. London: Smith, Elder, 1898.

McGrew, Roderick E. *Encyclopedia of Medical History*. New York: McGraw-Hill, 1985.

McNeal, Violet. *Four White Horses and a Brass Band*. Garden City: Doubleday, 1947.

Maehle, Andreas-Holger. *Drugs on Trial: Experimental Pharmacology and Therapeutic Innovation in the Eighteenth Century*. Clio Medica 53. Amsterdam: Rodopi, 1999.

Martineau, Harriet. *Harriet Martineau's Autobiography*. Vol. I. Boston: J. R. Osgood, 1877.

Molloy, J. Fitzgerald, ed. *Memoirs of Mary Robinson*. London: Gibbings, 1895.

Moore, Doris L. *Ada Countess of Lovelace*. London: John Murray, 1977.

Moore, Thomas. *The Life, Letters and Journals of Lord Byron*. London: John Murray, 1901 (1st published 1829).

Morgagni, Giambattista. *The Clinical Consultations of Giambattista Morgagni*. Trans. S. Jarcho. Boston: Francis A. Countway Library of Medicine, 1984.

Motion, Andrew. *Wainewright the Poisoner*. London: Faber & Faber, 2000.

Mudge, Bradford Keyes. *Sara Coleridge, A Victorian Daughter*. New Haven: Yale Univ. Press, 1989.

Nostrums and Quackery. 2 vols. Chicago: American Medical Assoc., 1911, 1921.

Oleson, Charles W. *Secret Nostrums and Systems of Medicine*. Chicago: Oleson, 1892.

Oliver, N. T. *Lee's Priceless Recipes*. Chicago: Laird & Lee, 1895.

"Opium." In *Encyclopædia Britannica*. Vol. XVII. Philadelphia: J. M. Stoddart, 1884.

Orieux, Jean. *Voltaire*. Trans. B. Bray and H. R. Lane. New York: Doubleday, 1979 (1st published in French).

Ovid. *Metamorphoses*. Trans. H. Gregory. New York: Viking, 1958.

Pachter, Henry M. *Paracelsus: Magic into Science*. New York: Henry Schuman, 1951.

Packard, Francis R. *The Life and Times of Pare: 1510–1590*. New York: Paul B. Hoeber, 1976.

Pagel, Walter. *Paracelsus*. Basel: Karger, 1982.

Palmer, Cynthia, and Michael Horowitz, eds. *Sisters of the Extreme: Women Writing on the Drug Experience*. Rochester, Vermont: Park Street, 2000.

Paracelsus. "The Diseases That Deprive Man of His Reason." *Four Treatises of Theophrastus von Hohenheim called Paracelsus*. Trans. G. Zilboorg. Ed. H. E. Sigerist. Baltimore: Johns Hopkins Univ. Press, 1941.

Parssinen, Terry M. *Secret Passions, Secret Remedies: Narcotic Drugs in British Society, 1820–1930*. Manchester: Manchester Univ. Press, 1983.

Pavel, Ernst. *The Poet Dying: Heinrich Heine's Last Years in Paris*. New York: Farrar, Straus & Giroux, 1995.

Peters, Catherine. *The King of Inventors: A Life of Wilkie Collins*. London: Martin Secker & Warburg, 1991.

Pharmacopœia Londinensis. London: Edwardus Griffin, 1618.

Pichois, Claude. *Baudelaire*. Trans. G. Robb. London: Hamish Hamilton, 1989 (1st published in French, 1987).

Pickering, George. *Creative Malady*. New York: Oxford Univ. Press, 1974.

Piozzi, Hester (Mrs. Thrale). *Glimpses of Italian Society*. London: Seeley, 1892.

Pliny, *The Natural History of Pliny, Book XX*. Vol. IV. Trans. J. Bostock and H. T. Riley. London: Henry G. Bohn, 1856.

Pollock, John. *Wilberforce*. New York: St. Martin's Press, 1977.

Pomet, Pierre. *A Compleat History of Druggs*. Vol. I. London, 1712 (1st published in French, 1694).

Porter, Roy. *The Greatest Benefit to Mankind*. New York: W. W. Norton, 1997.

Proust, Marcel. *Marcel Proust: Letters to His Mother*. Trans. G. D. Painter. London: Rider, 1956.

Psalmanazar, George. *Memoirs of ****, Commonly known by the Name of George Psalmanazar*. 2nd ed. London, 1765.

Quella-Villéger, Alain. *Le cas Farrère*. Paris: Presses de la Renaissance, 1989.

Rabbe, Alphonse. *Album d'un pessimiste*. Paris: Les Presses Françaises, 1924 (1st published 1835).

Raynaud, Maurice. *Les Médecins au temps de Molière*. Paris: Didier, 1863.

Richardson, Joseph G. *Medicology: or Home Encyclopedia of Health*. New York: University Medical Society, 1903.

Rousseau, Jean-Jacques. *The Confessions of Jean Jacques Rousseau*. Vol. I. Great Britain: n.p., 1904.

Seaman, Valentine. *An Inaugural Dissertation on Opium*. Philadelphia, 1792.

Secret Remedies. London: British Medical Assoc., 1909.

Sheaffer, Louis. *O'Neill: Son and Playwright*. Boston: Little, Brown, 1968.

Squire, Peter. *Squire's Companion*. London: J. & A. Churchill, 1908.

Steegmuller, Francis. *A Woman, A Man, and Two Kingdoms*. New York: Alfred A. Knopf, 1991.

Sterne, Madeleine B. *Louisa May Alcott*. New York: Random House, 1986.

Summerson, John. *Sir Christopher Wren*. London: Collins, 1953.

Sydenham, Thomas. *The Works of Thomas Sydenham, M. D.* London: Sydenham Society, 1858 (1st published 1680, 1682).

Tailhade, Laurent. *Les « Commérages » de Tybalt*. Paris: Collections «Les Proses », 1914.

———. *La « Noire idole » : Étude sur la morphinomanie*. Paris: Léon Vanier, 1907.

Terry, Charles, and Mildred Pellens. *The Opium Problem*. New York: Bureau of Social Hygiene, 1928.

Thurman, Judith. *Secrets of the Flesh: A Life of Colette*. New York: Alfred A. Knopf, 1999.

Trease, George E. *Pharmacy in History*. London: Baillière, Tindall & Cox, 1964.

Tuchman, Barbara. *The Proud Tower*. New York: Macmillan, 1962.

Wallace, A. H. *Guy de Maupassant*. Boston: Twayne, 1973.

Walsh, John. *Strange Harp, Strange Symphony: The Life of Francis Thompson*. New York: Hawthorn Books, 1967.

Watson, Gilbert. *Theriac and Mithridatium*. London: Wellcome Historical Medical Library, 1966.

Wilde, Oscar. "Pen, Poison and Ink." In *Intentions*. New York: Modern Library, 1920 (1st published 1891).

Wilson, Daniel. *Chatterton*. London: Macmillan, 1869.

Winter, William. *Old Friends*. New York: Moffat, Yard, 1909.

Wootton, A. C. *Chronicles of Pharmacy*. 2 vols. London: Macmillan, 1910.

Wordsworth, Dorothy. *The Grasmere Journals*. Ed. P. Woof. Oxford: Oxford Univ. Press, 1991.

Young, George. *A Treatise on Opium, Founded upon Practical Observations*. London, 1753.

Young, James H. *American Health Quackery*. Princeton: Princeton Univ. Press, 1992.

———. *The Toadstool Millionaires: A Social History of Patent Medicines*. Princeton: Princeton Univ. Press, 1961.

Yvorel, Jean-Jacques. *Les Poisons de l'esprit: drogues et drogués au XIXe siècle*. Paris: Quai Voltaire, 1992.

Fiction

Alcott, Louisa May. "A Marble Woman." In *Plots and Counterplots*. Ed. M. Stern. New York: William Morrow, 1976 (1st published 1865).

Balzac, Honoré de. "L'Opium." In *Œuvres diverses*. Vol. II. Eds. P.-G. Castex, R. Chollet, R. Guise, and C. Guise. Paris: Gallimard, 1996 (1st published 1830).

Brontë, Anne. *The Tenant of Wildfell Hall*. Oxford: Oxford Univ. Press, 1992 (1st published 1848).

Brontë, Charlotte. *Villette*. Harmondsworth: Penguin, 1985 (1st published 1853).

Buglakov, Mikhail. "Morphine." In *A Country Doctor's Notebook*. Trans. M. Glenny. London: Collins Harvill, 1975 (1st published 1925–27).

Byron, Lord. "To M.S.G." In *The Works of Lord Byron*. Paris: A. & W. Galignani, 1828.

Coleridge, Sara. "Poppies." In *Pretty Lessons in Verse*. London, J. W. Parker, 1834.

Collins, Wilkie. *Armadale*. New York: Peter Fenelon Collier, 1866.

———. *The Moonstone*. New York: Doubleday, 1946 (1st published 1868).

———. *No Name*. Harmondsworth: Penguin, 1994 (1st published 1862).

Daudet, Alphonse. *L'Évangéliste*. Paris: Flammarion, 1935 (1st published 1883).

———. *Sapho*. Paris: Flammarion, n.d. (1st published 1884).

Daudet, Léon. *La Lutte*. Paris: Flammarion, 1935 (1st published 1907).

Diver, Maud. *The Great Amulet*. Edinburgh: Blackwood & Sons, 1913.

Dubut de Laforest, Jean-Louis. *Morphine*. Paris: E. Dentu, 1891.

Dumas, Alexandre. *The Count of Monte Cristo*. Oxford: Oxford Univ. Press, 1990 (1st published in French, 1844–46).

Eliot, George. *Middlemarch*. New York: Modern Library, 1994 (1st published 1871–72).

Galdós, Benito Pérez. *Fortunata and Jacinta*. Trans. L. Clark. Harmondsworth: Penguin, 1973 (1st published in Spanish, c. 1890).

Garth, Samuel. *The Dispensary*. Dublin, 1725.

Gaskell, Elizabeth C. *Mary Barton*. London: Smith, Elder, 1906 (1st published 1848).

Halliday, Brett. *Counterfeit Wife*. New York: Dell, 1947.

Hammett, Dashiell. *The Dain Curse*. London:

Cassell, 1974 (1st published 1929).

———. *Red Harvest*. New York: Alfred A. Knopf, 1965 (1st published 1929).

Harlowe, Reginald. *Le Morphinomane assassin*. Bruxelles: Éditions Harlowe, n.d.

Heine, Heinrich. *The Complete Poems of Heinrich Heine*. Ed. and trans. H. Draper. Boston: Suhrkamp/Insel, 1982.

Huxley, Aldous. *Antic Hay*. Harmondsworth: Penguin, 1948 (1st published 1923).

Keats, John. "Ode to a Nightingale" and "The Eve of St Agnes." In *The Poetical Works of John Keats*. London: E. Moxon, Son, 1871.

London, Jack. *The Little Lady of the Big House*. New York: Macmillan, 1916.

Molière. *The Imaginary Invalid*. Adapted by Miles Malleson. London: Samuel French, 1959.

O'Neill, Eugene. *Long Day's Journey into Night*. New Haven: Yale Univ. Press, 1956.

Rowell, Earle Albert. *Dope Adventures of David Dare*. Nashville, TN: Southern Publishing Assoc., 1937.

Sand, George. *Valentine*. Trans. G. B. Ives, 1902. Chicago: Academy, 1995 (1st published in French, 1832).

Saussay, Victorien du. *La Morphine*. Paris: Albert Méricant, n.d.

Shelley, Mary. *Frankenstein*. Harmondsworth: Penguin, 1994 (1st published 1818).

Sinclair, Upton. *The Jungle*. New York: Barnes & Noble, 1995 (1st published 1906).

Smith, Charlotte. "Ode to the Poppy." In *Desmond*. Vol. III. London, 1792.

Souvestre, Pierre, and Marcel Allain. *Le Cercueil vide*. In *Fantômas*. Vol. II. Paris: Robert Laffont, 1988 (1st published 1913).

Stendhal. *The Charterhouse of Parma*. Trans. M. Mauldon. Oxford: Oxford Univ. Press, 1997 (1st published in French, 1839).

Stoker, Bram. *Dracula*. New York: Doubleday, n.d. (1st published 1897).

Stowe, Harriet Elizabeth Beecher. *Uncle Tom's Cabin*. London: J. M. Dent, 1909 (1st published 1852).

Thackeray, William M. *Vanity Fair*. 3 vols. New York: Charles Scribner's Sons, 1903 (1st published 1847).

Verne, Jules. "À la morphine." In *Poésies inédites*. Ed. C. Robin. Paris: Le cherche midi, 1989.

Yonge, Charlotte M. *The Three Brides*. London: Macmillan, 1850.

Periodicals

"Accidental Poisoning." In *Illustrated London News*. 3 December 1859.

Adams, Samuel Hopkins. "The Scavengers. The Great American Fraud." In *Collier's*. 22 September 1906.

Blair, William. "An Opium-Eater in America." In *The Knickerbocker*. July 1842.

"Coroners' Inquests." In *Illustrated London News*. 20 August, 17 September 1842.

"Death From Drinking Laudanum and Brandy." In *Illustrated London News*. 27 August 1859.

Derosne, Charles Louis. "Mémoire sur l'opium." In *Annales de chimie*. Paris: Fuchs, 30 Nivôse, an XI (1803).

"Epitome of News." In *Illustrated London News*. 3 June 1843.

"An Indianapolis woman . . ." In *Harper's Weekly*. 17 May 1873.

Kritikos, P. G., and S. P. Papadaki. "The History of the Poppy and of Opium and Their Expansion in Antiquity in the Eastern Mediterranean Area, Part I." In *Bulletin on Narcotics*. Vol. XIX, no. 3, July–September 1967.

"A 'Laudanum' District." In *Illustrated London News*. 27 March 1858.

"The Mayor and the Tenements." In *Harper's Weekly*. 15 October 1881.

"The Narcotics We Indulge In." In *Blackwood's*. November 1853.

"Opium-Eating." In *The Graphic*. 28 October 1876.

Pia, Pascal. "Les Paradis artificiels, de Baudelaire à Apollinaire." In *magazine littéraire*. November 1969.

"Samuel Taylor Coleridge." In *Quarterly Review*, reprinted in *Library Magazine*. c. 1890.

Séguin, Armand. "Sur l'opium." In *Annales de chimie*. Series I, vol. 92. Paris: Masson. 31 December 1814.

Sharkey, Seymour J. "Morphinomania." In *Nineteenth Century*, reprinted in *Library Magazine*. c. 1890.

"Suicide of Mr. Isaac Cohen." In *Illustrated London News*. 25 March 1843.

Weill, Paul B. "The Structure of Morphine." In *Bulletin on Narcotics*. Vol. II, no. 2, April 1950, 8–20.

Acknowledgements

Nick Bantock, for spotting the poem "Cocaine Lil and Morphine Sue"; Todd Belcher, for his indispensable assistance with photography and for the loan of the *Squire's Companion;* Ron Gordon of Found Bound Books in New York; Michael Thompson of Thompson Rare Books; Charlie Haynes, for the photocopy of Dr. John Leake's *Chronic Diseases of Women;* Ted Pappas of West Coast Estates; John Lieffering, for the opportunity to photograph items in his collection; Reg Daggitt, for allowing me to photograph his collection of books as well as the laudanum bottle; Colin Schebek and Kym Lobzun, for allowing me to photograph their collection; Blair Shakell, for the loan of *Needle* and *Marijuana Murders;* Maurice Spira, for allowing me to tromp through his garden; the Vancouver Police Historical Society & Centennial Museum, for allowing me to photograph newspaper clippings and police head shots; Joan Seidl, curator of history at the Vancouver Museum; Lee Perry, of the Woodward Biomedical Library, for her help with my research; John Barthel and Maryse Claude of Vintage Video in Toronto, for their help with special movie requests; Molly Munro, for the morphine bottle; Jean-Louis Dorricott, for the Rousseau reference; Sandra Fleming, for the tips on movies and objects; Maureen Nicholson, for her careful proofreading. Thanks as well to Doctor Andreas-Holger Maehle, Grevel Lindop, Theodore Roszak and D. L. Macdonald for their responses to my importuning letters. And to the many movie and literature buffs who suggested sources: thanks to you all.

Special thanks to Dr. James Dickie and Dr. Christian Fouanon, who have generously shared their opium interests and collections with me; to Nancy Flight, for her attentive editing; to Saeko Usukawa, for her incredible devotion to digging up obscure facts; and to David Gay, whose patience is unparalleled.

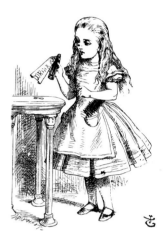

"Drink Me." Alice contemplates a bottle that contains a mysterious substance in Lewis Carroll's *Alice's Adventures in Wonderland.* Carroll's readers have long speculated about the contents of the bottle in Alice's hand. Some suggest that it contained an opiated drug that caused her to dream that she was alternatively shrinking and growing. Elsewhere in his tale, Carroll introduces a hookah-smoking caterpillar, a clearer reference to drugs, in this instance, hashish. London: Macmillan, 1911. Illustration by John Tenniel.

(US 1910); Turvey Treatment for Alcoholism and Narcomania (GB n.d.); Weatherby's Opium Antidote (US 1909).

Index